The Resilience Reflex

8 Keys to Transforming Barriers into Success in Life and Business

By

Zaheen Nanji

Emily,

You've got this!

ZN

The Resilience Reflex – 8 Keys to Transforming Barriers into Success in Life and Business

ISBN 978-0-9949224-0-3

Printed In Canada

Message from Zaheen Nanji and BONUS Gift Offer

Thank you for starting your journey toward a resilient life. This book was supposed to be my first book because I've wanted to share my message for a long time, but I wasn't ready. Instead, I published a short book on behavior weight loss first, which went on to win an award. I just didn't want to write a book about my story, but I wanted to provide the tools for others to overcome barriers, embrace change, and bounce back.

I hope you'll purchase your copy today and enjoy this BONUS gift immediately:

A workbook based on the 3-step system found in this book.

Visit http://www.zaheennanji.com/rrbook to access this BONUS gift now!

THE RESILIENCE REFLEX

WORKBOOK

3 Powerful Steps to Get Unstuck and Bounce Back

ZAHEEN NANJI

Introduction

Resiliency is something I started learning about at a very young age. My mother taught all of us children to work hard and to keep going whenever life knocked us around a bit. There were times I thought that my circumstances were going to keep me down forever. I developed a stutter around the age of five, and it almost kept me from my purpose and my passions. Thankfully, experiences I had and the people who surrounded me during my journey down life's pathway led me to embracing my fears and stepping into clarity and fulfillment.

I believe everyone can learn how to take what life gives them and learn how to turn their pain into purpose. I learned how to do this and it resulted in me—an ordinary South Asian girl who grew up in Africa and then moved to Canada—being able to thrive.

This book is broken into three parts because I wanted you to understand where I've been, the obstacles I have overcome, the lessons I've learned in the process, and the habits and beliefs I have developed in order to become resilient in life and business. The second part of the book gives you the eight keys to transform your barriers into success, and as you consciously practice and implement these keys, you will start noticing how easily you are able to get unstuck, problem solve, and move forward. The third part of this book gives you specific tools and a 3-step system to build your resilience muscle so you can make resilience your first reflex when faced with challenges.

I'm so grateful to:

My mother for instilling in me values and making me feel capable to do anything I set my mind to.

My husband, Badur, for being my support system and helping me fulfill my dreams.

My daughter, Arissa, for understanding the times that I had to lock myself in my office and write or travel, but yet encouraging me to do it.

My hope is that after reading this book, you will start using the methods and tools outlined in the book and become a resilient champion!

Zaheen Nanji

Table of Contents

Zaheen Nanji

PART 1 – The Road to Resiliency

Chapter 1

The Phone Call

In 1972, the president of Uganda, Idi Amin, expelled all South Asians from the country. Most moved to the UK, the United States, and Canada. However, my family lived in East Africa (made up of Uganda, Tanzania, and Kenya), in Kenya specifically, and after Amin's decree, most South Asians there and in Tanzania feared for their livelihood. In fact, in the 1980s and 90s, there was a mass movement of South Asians from East Africa to North America. Even now, there is violence in Kenya—from the bombing of the prestigious Westgate Mall in Nairobi in 2013, where my nephew almost lost his life, to the ongoing threats and gun shots in my home town of Mombasa. In addition, there are robberies nightly that sometimes turn out to be fatal. Not knowing what the future would bring in a place where stability was compromised, my parents took an opportunity to send my sisters and me to Canada in 1990.

"Mummy, I want to go to Toronto. All my friends are moving there, and I really feel there is nothing for me here," said my sister Nilufar, then 20. She had applied at the Canadian embassy, but her application was rejected.

"Can we apply for permanent residence visas as a family? We may get accepted," urged Nilufar. We were a family of eight; my parents ran a thriving bakery business and were not at all interested in moving to Canada. They simply couldn't imagine living in a country where it dropped to minus 30 degrees Celsius! But my parents submitted an application, and lo and behold, it was accepted.

"I really don't want to go," I overheard my mother confiding in her sister in our native language. "We're finally doing so well in the business and making more money than ever. How can I leave this and start all over again? I can't even speak English!"

"Guli," replied my aunt, "don't just think about you. There have been so many families applying for permanent residency in Canada and most are getting rejected. This is an opportunity for your children to get a better education and access to good health care. It's easier to get into university if they complete their schooling in Canada, and it will be cheaper than sending them to UK like most of us do. You are very lucky you got this opportunity."

Nilufar moved to Toronto, Ontario, while my sister, Zohreen, then 17, went to Edmonton, Alberta, to stay with my mother's older sister for a few months until my mom and I arrived. I was just 15 years old at the time.

The houses, yards, and gardens looked so pristine, just like in the movies. *Why do people complain about the cold weather? It's beautiful here,* I thought, only to realize that this great weather lasts just a few months out of the year.

One beautiful Sunday afternoon, I couldn't believe my eyes as Zohreen started to mow my aunt's lawn—we had never done that in Kenya! We didn't have lawns.

"What are you doing?" I asked.

While my sister mowed, my cousin interjected, "You both have to learn how to do this. There are no servants and nannies here like you have in Kenya. You have to do it all yourself, so why not start now?"

My mom seemed incapable of staying anywhere for longer than three weeks, so as soon as she found an apartment and settled us in, she left for Mombasa to go back to my younger brothers. She had opened a bank account and though I don't remember much about the money situation, I do recall that Zohreen handled most of that, and she even found herself a job at McDonald's before I had arrived, on the advice of my cousin.

As she worked during that summer, I was left alone in the apartment. I loved the feel of carpet all over the place, something we never had in our house in Kenya. I was amazed that there were machines that could wash and dry our clothes, but I had no idea how to use them until I asked my aunt to show me. The best part was having a machine to wash the dishes; no wonder they didn't have servants and nannies to do the job. They had machines!

One day, I was home alone, waiting for my sister to return from work. There was no furniture in the living room, nothing but the television and the telephone. I loved watching the programs on TV, and there were so many channels to choose from, unlike Kenya where we only had five channels, and most of them were in the native language, Kiswahili. In Kenya, with a family of eight and living in an enclosed community, I was never home alone. There was always someone around. I didn't like being home alone and I was scared. Having the TV on loud, so I could hear it in any every room of the apartment, helped calm my nerves.

Suddenly, I was startled by the phone ringing (this was well before caller I.D.) *Oh no!* I thought to myself. *Do I answer the phone? Who could be calling? I really don't want to answer the phone!* I felt my heart thumping in my chest and my hands getting cold and clammy. My throat tightened up as I slowly reached to answer the phone, but I quickly pulled my hand back because it was shaking.

I wish someone else would answer the phone! I scream (in my head). Then the phone stopped ringing. *Phew! I am glad I did not answer that,* I said silently to myself and sat down on the carpeted living room floor. A minute hadn't gone by, and it rang again! *Trringtrring! Trring rring!* My throat tightened again, and I tried gulping several times and breathing, but to no avail. *What if it's Zohreen calling?* I thought. As I picked up the receiver, it felt like 100 pounds. I put it slowly to my ear.

"H–h-hello?" I said in a soft voice while the TV played in the background. A gentleman's voice came on, but I didn't understand a word, and he was talking too fast. I wanted to tell him to slow down so I could understand, but I couldn't even speak a word. I couldn't breathe, my chest was tight, and my hand was clenched tightly over the phone while I wrapped the opposite arm around my legs to bring my knees to my chest.

There was a pause on the other end and then, "Hello?" he said. "Hello? Are you there?" he repeated.

"Y-y-yes," I replied, and he started rambling on again. The only thing I heard him say was, "I am asking…" Then came another pause, and I knew he wanted me to answer. I took a deep breath and quickly said the only words I could manage: "I can't hear you."

So, he got louder! But all I heard was the TV noise and my heart thumping. I could sense frustration in his voice, and I felt sorry for him.

"I am not doing this on purpose; if only you knew why I can't say what I want to say," I felt like telling him. Before he finished speaking, I hung up. The tension immediately released from my throat and chest, but still I stared at the phone like it was a snake about to bite.

The phone rang again. *Trringtrring! Trringtrring!* I picked up the receiver and put it to my ear to hear the same gentleman; this time he was yelling at me, but all I could hear him say was, "Turn off the TV!" Then he continued on even more loudly and more frustrated than before. The more frustrated he became, the tighter my throat became, and I couldn't utter a word. By then, my whole body was shaking and I hung up—again.

I didn't want the phone to ring so I pulled the cord out of the wall and turned off the TV. I curled up again so scared, still shaking, and then I cried. "I am so stupid, I am so stupid," I said, crying and banging my forehead on my knees. *How will I make my life in a new country when I feel so dumb and helpless? I can't even read a sentence or order a meal, let alone answer the phone! Why is it that every time I want to say something, I have to think of what words I can say and what words I need to avoid?*

"I'm not going to live here; I am going back to Kenya. I can't survive here!" I wiped my tears away. "Other kids will make fun of me in school, and I will hate it." However, in the back of my mind, I knew there was no going back.

I could feel every cell in my body screaming, "I wish I didn't stutter!" With a stutter that controlled my life, how could I expect to survive the next few years in high school?

We string words to create dialogue, to have meaningful conversations, to inspire others with a moving speech, and all of these have two things in common: communication and creating relationships. The average person may not think twice when she opens her mouth to have a conversation; the words just flow out. That's not the case for a person who stutters. A person who stutters has a different experience, because the words don't just flow out. Speech tends to have involuntary disruptions that have been labeled as blocks, prolongations, and repetitions. Imagine a broken car that is a wreck and is still being driven. It resists moving, sputters, jerks, revs up, sighs, jerks again, sputters. It's the same for someone who stutters. For some reason, people who stutter hate speaking on the phone, maybe because the words take so long to come out that they assume the person on the other end becomes impatient. As I look back on this incident, I realize that most of us get stuck on some problem and don't know how to become unstuck. I think what was most traumatizing for me was the tone and frustration I heard in the man's voice. He may have felt he wasn't being heard or understood. Yet, I didn't know that then; all I could see was my negative future ahead of me.

Whenever I re-play this incident in my head, I ask myself, "What could I have done differently?" Could I have turned down the volume of the television or completely turned it off? Could I have asked him to slow down so I could understand him better? I was so focused on NOT stuttering when answering the phone that the other ideas never occurred to me.

However, had I known then what I know now, I'd have focused on becoming unstuck from that state of "not stuttering" and focused instead on what I wanted.

I wanted to speak on the phone with authenticity and to be relaxed instead of agitated. I wanted to focus on what he was saying rather than focusing on myself. I wanted to breathe and to use my voice. I just wanted to be me instead of someone hiding behind this mask of perfectionism. Fear was my best friend and my worst enemy—it kept me safe from being embarrassed and feeling vulnerable, but it also kept me from the things I really wanted to do. All my life I had lived in conflict because I felt I had to be perfect and to hide my stutter so that no one could see the real me, but the perfect mask was slowly being torn away.

It's amazing how an inanimate object like the phone had so much control over me. Instead of looking at the opportunity I had to enhance my life and education, I could only see the negative aspects and how this new life was going to ruin my mask of perfection. *How would my classmates treat me in this new world if they found out that I stutter? Would I even have friends or would they call me a freak?* These thoughts consumed me, and I began to feel worse and to have crazy images in my head. This is where most people get stuck, and so did I. Negative thoughts and feelings consume our life and block our vision of what is possible. In addition, negative thoughts and feelings keep guiding our behavior in a way that invites more negativity and chaos.

Instead of asking, "HOW can I solve this problem," we tend to focus on, "WHY is this happening to me?" Interestingly, in Kenya, I had learned how to solve the problem by substituting words, breathing deeply before I spoke, and even completely avoiding speaking situations that terrified me. But that only solved half of the problem. Life is a learning journey; we never stop learning and developing skills. Making a habit of asking the right questions can help us get unstuck from a problem that could be taking us down a path that leads nowhere. At that time, I failed to realize that I needed additional skills to conquer my fear of stuttering, but I learned that lesson later on when faced with another obstacle.

In this chapter alone, you will find there isn't just one obstacle. There I was, a 15-year-old girl who had come to a new country, new culture, and a new way of living with her 17-year-old sister, who was also going through her own inner fears related to fitting in. On top of being in a new world without our parents, we also had to be responsible for all sorts of things, such as paying the bills, grocery shopping, cooking, going to school, and completing our homework. But I survived; I overcame these obstacles and I became resilient.

Chapter 2

Revelation

In today's world, I hear organizations and individuals say that they are doing more with less, or they have too much on their plate. In fact, the "S" word is used 24/7, and the word I am referring to is *stress!* The HeartMath Institute in California describes stress in this way: "Stress is a perception. Stress occurs when an individual's perception of pressure or challenge exceeds his/her perceived ability to cope" (Spring 2006 Newsletter from Institute of HeartMath).

What this means is that most of us blame our external environment for the stress in our lives, but stress is actually caused by how we choose to react to a situation. The World Health Organization has estimated that by the year 2020, clinical depression will outrank cancer and be the second leading disease after heart disease. It's only after operating a wellness centre that I realized the majority of our clients who have suffered a trauma or have demanding jobs or toxic work environments are on anti-depressants. I was surprised when a client whose mother had passed away was prescribed anti-depressants to help her grieve. Managing one's emotional reaction to pressure, challenge, or conflict is key to managing wellness without the use of drugs.

Our response to stress is similar to our response to fear—it's meant to keep us safe from harm. When faced with fear, the body produces extra cortisol and adrenaline so that we can get into the fight or flight reaction. Unfortunately, the body releases the same chemicals when we are stressed, but we don't use it for fight or flight; it simply goes nowhere and builds up in the body. This build up of cortisol results in symptoms like muscle tension, headaches, panic attacks, the common cold, or irritable bowel syndrome. If not taken care of, any of these problems can develop into chronic conditions. Our body sends us subtle signals and messages, yet most us either tend to ignore them or don't know HOW to deal with stress. Do you find yourself getting irritable, angry, or exhausted when you have taken on too much or have been plugging through day after day? These are the first signs of burnout.

You don't realize that your body is smarter than you think. Even though we produce chemicals when we perceive stress, we can also produce the endorphins, which give a natural high and relax the nervous and immune systems. Numerous studies have shown that incorporating positive emotions and learning to let go releases endorphins and balances out the system. In this digital world, information is like an open tap of water; it just keeps pouring out and it can get overwhelming. But we can control this overload of information and this need to know and do it all by just practicing to turn our body's energy system off every once in a while. One trait of successful and resilient individuals is they take a break from digital information on weekends and completely unplug during holidays.

I come from a family of entrepreneurs, and I married into a family of entrepreneurs. I have witnessed it and done it myself; we keep working and wish we had more hours in the day to just complete a task so we can get ahead, or take on another merger, or introduce another idea. I have extended family members who make millions but suffer from panic attacks; I also have extended family members who work long hours in a day and suffer from chronic health issues.

One afternoon when I was five years old, I was playing with my toys in the bedroom I shared with three of my siblings. My mother was reading her favourite magazine, *Woman's Own*, when there was a knock at the door. Our door was always open when our parents' were home, and I heard unfamiliar voices greet my mother. When I came out of the bedroom, I saw that it was the parents of a couple of my classmates.

"We were just wondering what you thought of your daughter's report card," one of the women said with a smile as she sat down on the couch.

I darted behind the four-foot wall separating the living room and the dining room. A visit from unexpected guests who wanted to talk about my report card couldn't be good.

When I peeked around the corner, I saw my mother smiling proudly. "I was very impressed with it and also with the very nice remarks from the teacher."

The smell of curry wafted from the kitchen, and I smiled to myself, knowing I had made my mother proud.

"Some of our children have done really well, and the school board feels that these children are so smart that they could easily skip grade 1 and go into grade 2." My mother seemed curious and yet confused. "Your daughter, Zaheen, is one of them," said the parent. My mother's expression again went from a proud momma in one minute to a concerned momma the next minute. My mother was speechless. As they continued to convince my mother that they had already spoken to the other parents, and the board was willing to pilot this project, I remember being very scared and nervous. A part of me wanted to reach out and say no and tell my mother not to go ahead because I wanted to stay with the rest of my friends in the same class. A part of me felt like I couldn't say anything because I was supposed to listen to my parents, and they had expectations of me, and my opinion didn't matter. One of the parents asked my mother, "Will you let Zaheen be a part of this project?" my mother hesitated. I felt like I was hanging onto a rope for dear life, too scared to look down. I could see her feeling pressured to make a decision, having a lot of concern for me, but yet wondering, *May be my daughter is capable.* I heard her say, "Yes," and it felt like the rope let go.

This challenge exceeded my ability to cope, and that is when *the symptom*—stuttering—began. For the longest time, I didn't know why I stuttered or how it began, but I figured it out in 2009 when I was in my master practitioner neuro linguistic programming (NLP) class. NLP is also known as the study of human behaviour. During one of our classes, my colleague Xavier and I were partnered to try timeline therapy. In this exercise, we had to walk across an imaginary straight line from birth to present and notice how some of the events in our life had shaped our future; then, we were to consider the lessons brought forth from those events.

"Okay Xavier, I'm going first," I stated as I started walking very slowly as though I was on a tight rope. After a few seconds, I stopped, and Xavier asked, "Do you sense something?"

"Yes, I've always wondered why I stuttered or how I started, and I get the feeling it's around the ages of five to seven—right around where I have stopped. This is so creepy."

"Take a moment and remember the first time you think you started stuttering or what caused you to start stuttering," Xavier prompted gently.

In NLP, we were taught to acknowledge any images or thoughts that came up for us because those are the answers we could be seeking. As soon as Xavier asked that question, an image of me watching my mother from the corner of the four-foot wall came up. I stopped breathing, and time came to a halt. I was back at the scene, and my throat tightened up again.

Xavier noticed my expression and the physiological signs. He gently touched my shoulder and said, "Breathe and take a step away from the timeline." As soon as I did that, I took in a deep breath and sighed. I explained what I had seen, and we decided to work on it some more.

Xavier asked me, "What was the positive intention behind your symptom of stuttering; what was the gain behind this experience?" I had never thought of stuttering as a symptom and being a gain for me because I hated that I stuttered. I answered, but it wasn't the adult me answering; I felt like my little self at the age of five saying, "I did not want to go to grade 2, and if there is something wrong with me, then I will be able to stay in grade 1."

Our core beliefs involving love and security are formed in childhood between the ages of three and eight because they are linked to survival. Peter Halligan, a psychologist at Cardiff University, says, "A belief is a mental architecture of how we interpret the world." As human beings, we make meaning out of everything, and these meanings lead to thoughts and beliefs that guide our behaviour. I attached various meanings to this incident at the age of five: I am smart; I am different; I can't fail. My parents have expectations of me, and I can't let them down; my opinion doesn't matter; I can't say what I want because I'll get into trouble. I have to work hard to catch up to grade 2 because they think I am smart.

I became an over-achiever and worked hard to catch up. These beliefs helped me throughout my life, but they also caused problems with my mental and emotional health. I didn't know how to stop or delegate or work in harmony. Instead, I felt I had to make it work and prove that I was capable, and in the process, I burned out. There were times that I'd take on so much because I thought I could do it, but overtime, it became overwhelming, and still I didn't complain because I felt I had to be strong. Twice, I ended up crying on the dining table while having tea with my husband, Badur, and the second time, he told me what I needed to hear.

"Why are you crying?"

"I'm just so tired, so tired," I sobbed and continued. "I work full-time, I help at the wellness centre, and I'm working toward making professional speaking my career, and I don't even have time for me. I like getting my nails done like other women; I want to go to Mexico like other people, but we just haven't had the time. I'm so exhausted."

"You know what your problem is? You want to do everything," he blurted out. "You can't do it all. Become an expert in one thing and focus on that. I don't need you at the wellness centre every day, but pick two days you want to be there. And get your manicure because only you can make yourself feel good; no one else can." I looked at Badur in amazement and kept sobbing, knowing that he was so right. He continued, "Zaheen, most of all, you need to decide what you want to do because you are dabbling in too many areas."

The people who care about us the most will tell us what we need to hear because they know us better than anyone else. Badur and I continued talking about how I could delegate and who I could get help from to work toward my passion and help me figure out my area of expertise. During this time, he also mentioned behaviours that I was expressing that were leading toward burnout.

"How come you didn't tell me this before?" I said as I gently slapped him on his chest.

"You were already crabby, and I didn't want to add more fuel to the fire. Now that you have let it out, I feel you are ready to listen," he answered. And then he said, "I've noticed you start getting irritable first, like we are in your way. Then you get angry or upset easily. For example, if I ask you something, you get upset at me for no reason. This goes on for days, and it's difficult to make you aware that you are behaving this way," explained Badur.

"You know, hon, it's not that I like being this way. I become more conscious of it when it's too late, like today, and I have to work on breaking this pattern. I have to recognize these symptoms earlier, and you just made me aware of my pattern."

We are so used to behaving in a certain manner that it becomes our default behaviour in a particular situation. These default behaviours are ingrained in our brain as neural pathways and are difficult to change unless one becomes consciously aware of them or someone makes us aware of them. However, the choices one makes after becoming aware are more important.

The first step to change is noticing how our senses work. My pattern consisted of the following:

1. Taking on too much and then becoming overwhelmed. Here I noticed that I'd create visual images of mountains of paperwork and housework (sensory pattern – visual -V).

2. Feeling irritable and angry. Here I'd start to doubt that I could get the work done and then the fear of failure seeped in. I didn't like feeling negative, so I'd take it out on my family (sensory pattern – kinesthetic -K).

3. Exhaustion and negative self-talk. I'd keep going and ignore the gremlin, but in the end, I'd get exhausted, cry, and wish things were different (sensory pattern – kinesthetic/auditory - A).

The sequence of the pattern is visual (V), kinesthetic (K), and auditory (A).

I consciously started to change this default pattern of taking on too much. Now when I get an idea or a new task comes on my plate, I choose to do the following:

1. Ask myself, "Can I take it on? What else do I have on my calendar?" I visualize my calendar to see what other projects I have and to check if I have the time. If I know I don't have the time to take it on and/or if I know it is not a good fit for me, I pass (sensory pattern – auditory/visual).

2. While I'm working through the first step, I'm also checking my feelings and listening to my intuition (kinesthetic).

The sequence of the pattern is now auditory (A), visual (V), and kinesthetic (K). As I started to consciously practice this pattern, I realized how much more freedom I had. In fact, in one year, I delegated tasks, such as social media and marketing, to a team member; I hired a coach to help me figure out my area of expertise so I could focus on one message and get really good at it; and I hired a virtual assistant to manage my queries and complete simple tasks. I now take time to meditate at 4:45 a.m., respond to inquiries and write my blogs between 5 and 7 a.m., and pamper myself with a massage and manicure once a month.

Change is inevitable, and if anyone says to you that you have to have balance, you must know that there is no such thing. Like my friend Terry Wildemann says, "When people talk about work-life balance, the scale is stagnant and nothing is happening which could lead to inaction. What we need is work-life harmony, where we can flow in and out of different areas in our life and at the same time refocus and rejuvenate."

Do you recognize any of the symptoms of stress in you? Do you recall the last time you were exhausted or overworked? Is there a pattern that you can describe with your senses or even a pattern of procrastination, such as waiting to get the work done when the deadline approaches? With the plethora of messages we get through email and social media, do you have a pattern of wasting time and reading every post or e-newsletter?

Notice the beliefs you have formed about events that have occurred in the past and how they guide your behaviour. Stuttering was my survival mechanism in case I couldn't cope, but then it became ingrained as a neural pathway, and at the same time excellence became my coping mechanism. Both of these mechanisms caused conflict throughout my life because I wasn't sure who I wanted to be or what I wanted. I'm still learning more about myself every day.

Devote time to take inventory of your life and force yourself to do things that matter to you most. Delegate tasks that others can do efficiently and be very aware of your primary senses—the images you visualize, the things you say to yourself, and the feelings you vibrate; ensure they are positive. New changes take time to implement and embracing change takes practice.

In 2011, I visited my mother in Kenya. We had a deep conversation about thoughts, emotions, and life in general, when I asked her, "Mom, when did I start stuttering?"

She replied, "When I made the decision that you could skip grade 1." She continued, "Zaheen, I am sorry that because of my decision, you had to miss out on a normal childhood, and I know there were times you hated yourself for not being able to talk or do things you wanted. I hope you can forgive me."

"Mom, I never blamed you for that decision; you had the best intentions for me. To tell you the truth, feeling like I didn't have a voice was the worst experience at that time, but looking back, I realize that I wouldn't be the person I am today without that experience."

Chapter 3

Embracing Change

In this day and age, change is inevitable. Technological changes, new product developments and marketing, changes in the global economy, and personal life changes or career changes happen all around us. The universe and our human history are great teachers of change and resiliency, yet we fear change because we are unsure of what lies on the other side. We start doubting our capability to cope, and we end up resisting change. Resilient individuals cope better with change, even though they have fears about it just like others do. However, instead of doubting themselves and resisting change, they get curious.

Curiosity is borne from our attitude, and psychologists define attitude as a learned tendency to evaluate things in a certain way. When resilient individuals approach a difficult situation, they have an attitude of being curious, patient, and optimistic, thereby diminishing fear of change.

Attitudes are also formed as a direct result of our experiences, values, and beliefs, and these guide our behaviours and actions toward a response. You've heard people say, "Have a positive attitude," but what does that mean? When I research resiliency in individuals, I have found that positive attitude encompasses the following traits that are guided by values and beliefs:

- Creative and solution-thinking
- Hope and gratitude
- Expectation of some success
- Lessons from setbacks
- Belief in their capability
- Flexibility and fulfilment
- Networking

These traits are similar to that of a scientist, aren't they? A scientist has to be creative, expect some success, repeat experiments after some setbacks and lessons, and believe that he or she can be successful in creating a new invention. If we were to approach a difficult situation or a major change in our life, work, or business like a scientist, would that make life a little easier?

One common question posed to me by clients and friends is, "How did two teenage girls manage living halfway across the world in a new society and culture without their parents?" My first answer would have been, "We just did." I always wondered why people in North America found it surprising and intriguing that my sister and I took care of ourselves.

Looking back, I believe that our upbringing and positive attitude toward life and opportunity prepared us for the new challenge. The decision to send us to Canada so that we could get access to a better education and health care was ingrained in us as the "opportunity of a lifetime." Thinking otherwise was not an option.

From the time I could remember, my parents owned a bakery business, and their day started at 4:30 am and ended at 5 pm. As the fourth of six children, my older siblings would wake us up, and we'd help each other get ready.

"It's six o' clock; wake up!" Nilufar, our older sister, would yell out from her bunk bed that was across from my bunk bed. Four of us slept in one bedroom. *Cukurooku, Cukurooku!* We'd hear the rooster wake us up, too, and we'd hurry to put on our uniforms that were hung neatly ironed in our shared closets.

"We can't afford to miss the school bus today because no one's here to take us to school," reminded Nilufar as we'd hurriedly brush our teeth and groom ourselves using one shared bathroom and sink.

"Chai is in the thermos and there's bread, butter, and jam on the table. Start spreading your own bread and pour chai in your cup." As soon as we'd finished eating breakfast, we'd run out the door toward the red and green school bus at 7:30 am; this was our routine every day, which made us independent from a very young age.

My faith is a large part of who I am and how I identify myself. We'd pray at home instead of going to *Jamatkhana* (place of worship) because mom wanted us to complete our homework and go to bed early. Our prayers were usually recited in a congregation out aloud, and one person recited the prayers while the rest listened in silence.

"Okay, come on all, it's 7 o'clock. Let's sit down in the living room and start our prayers," mom said aloud one day. "Who's going to say the first prayer?" she asked.

"I'm not saying it. Why can't Zaheen say it today? She doesn't have to say it; how come?" retorted one of my siblings. I looked at my mother with desperation. With my eyes, I pleaded: *please don't make me say it.*

She looked at me with concern and compassion, and said, "It's only your family here, and you have to start practicing. Take your time and recite as much as you can."

"Can I just recite the first two verses only?" I asked softly, knowing that my siblings would never tease me about my stutter, but I didn't want to take up so much time reciting prayers and for them to think: *How much time will she take?*

"Yes, then next time you can go up to three verses and so on, okay *beta* (my child)?"

I took a deep breath, looked at my siblings for support, and started. I stuttered, and I sputtered, and I had blocks on various sounds, but I got through it. A part of me knew that I couldn't avoid public speaking all my life, but then I became aware of how my mother used this time to instill in me beliefs about my abilities, and she instilled in us the attitude of gratitude. We'd always end our prayers with a feeling of gratitude and hope.

The first day we arrived at my aunt's house in North Edmonton, Canada, I noticed my sister washed the dishes after supper and my cousin swept the kitchen floor. The next day, my mother and her sister were baking and talking about their childhood days while I listened, and at the same time, I longed to be home in a familiar environment. Lunch time rolled around and as we finished our meal, mom whispered to me, "Go wash the dishes." I looked at her bewildered because first of all, I hadn't washed the dishes in a long time, and I was worried I'd break a lot of dishes, and secondly, I wondered if there was a different method of washing dishes in Canada.

"No," I whispered back.

"Bai, Zaheen is going to wash the dishes. Can you show her how you want her to wash them?" Mom said to her sister. My eyes widened, and I started to walk toward the heap of dishes in the kitchen sink.

"I washed the dishes today and mopped the floor," I whispered to my sister when she came home from her job that evening.

"Get used to it. This is just the beginning. Here you have to work and then come home, cook, and do all the chores yourself," Zohreen replied.

The next day, I begged mom to take me back.

"Zaheen, listen to me," Mom said, "It's difficult for me to leave you both here. It hurts me that I will not see you every day. I don't want to do this either, but we have this opportunity, and I can't let it get away from you without even trying."

She continued, "I have taught you a lot about this world, and you both have to be careful, but at the same time, I have also taught you how to be responsible and independent young women, isn't that correct?" Mom asked for a confirmation.

"Yes," I nodded.

"We are doing this for your future, and I know it's a big change for you, but have faith and be strong. You have each

30

other, and you are both very smart and mature. I would not be doing this if I didn't think you were both capable," she stressed.

We moved into an apartment that was right next to my grandmother's sister, my grandaunt, and I felt less homesick because we could visit my grandaunt every day, and we'd go to *Jamatkhana*—our place of worship. A seven-minute drive with my grandaunt and her husband, going to our prayer house, and being around others who belong to the same faith helped alleviate the sadness I felt about being away from family.

As I was accustomed to tropical weather, the Canadian winters were completely unexpected. We had been warned by our relatives to be prepared for the cold snap, but since we had never experienced it, how could we really prepare for it? My granduncle took us to the Army & Navy Salvation store and bought us some winter jackets, gloves, and toques. The first time I put them on, I wondered how I could ever walk in them, but they were lifesavers because I had never experienced my fingers and toes freezing to a point that I couldn't feel them anymore until my first winter.

As months passed, I made friends in school and even took guitar classes. The feeling of being homesick slowly disappeared, and I was starting to enjoy my new life.

A lot of the skills I have now, I attribute to my mother. Even though I haven't spent as much time with her as my other siblings have, I'm told we are very much alike. I remember small behaviours my mother had from making to-do lists in the morning to cooking and multi-tasking in the evening.

"Mom, what do you write every morning?" I asked one Saturday morning while still in Mombasa, Kenya.

"I'm making a list for myself of things to do this weekend, and I'm making a list for the servants to complete some chores," she replied.

"This is similar to the lists of chores you make for us during our holidays, isn't it?" I asked.

"Yes. This list helps me stay organized, and I can manage myself and others better."

People who know me and have followed my journey often comment, "Zaheen, I don't know how you pull things off. You are such a busy lady! How do you do it?" They know that apart from being a mother and wife, I have worked a full time job, while simultaneously building and running two businesses—a wellness centre business with my husband and my professional speaking career. Furthermore, I have published an award-winning book and started my own internet TV show.

I'm not tooting my own horn. I'm only demonstrating that a person can achieve what he or she wants with the appropriate passion and drive. I had a great role model growing up, and I learned how to prioritize, manage time, and be responsible for my actions because afterwards, I could enjoy the rewards, and I looked forward to that.

My mentors, Kris and Tim Hallbom, taught me a lot about human behaviour, and one of the models they invented is called the Universal Cycles of Change (UCC) model that has seven phases of change. In their research, they found that our unconscious patterns are similar to the patterns we see in the environment. Therefore, if you have conscious awareness of this model and its seven phases, you will live a harmonious life where you are consistently getting what you want. I use this model every day in my life and business, and I have consistently gotten what I want. These seven phases are within all systems:

1. Creation. This phase is about new beginnings, new birth, or a new idea.
2. Growth. This phase is about growth and expansion.
3. Complexity to maturity. As a system begins to take shape and form, there comes a point when the system is in its steady state.

4. Turbulence. When a system keeps growing and becomes complex, turbulence sets in. This is considered feedback from the system that it can longer cope; it needs support.

5. Chaos. This phase sets in when the system starts to fall apart.

6. Releasing. This phase is about letting go of things that no longer serve you so the system can get back into balance.

7. Dormancy/mediation. This phase is about regaining harmony and ruminating over the lessons from previous phases, so you can start to create and grow again.

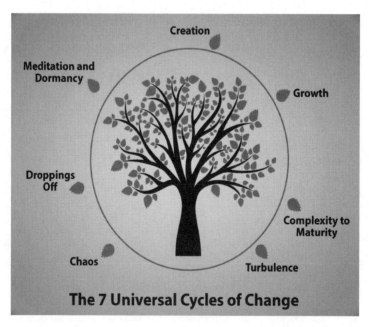

The 7 Universal Cycles of Change

All living systems in nature are in sync with this model, except for one living system—humans! We love hanging around the turbulence and chaos phase for a long time and we tend to resist change because of our fear of letting go. Assess different areas of your life from money matters to health, relationships to business and career. Are you experiencing chaos and turbulence in any of these areas of your life? Can you let go of one small aspect to regain balance? For example, I let go of watching late night television so I could wake up at 4:45 am to meditate and complete some tasks. Successful people are very much in tune with this model because they understand that when they let go, new opportunities can emerge.

*Model and photo courtesy of Tim and Kris Hallbom, NLP Institute of California

Chapter 4

Rewards

Chores are easier in North America than in Kenya, but why? Well, it is because there are machines to do the job for you. In Kenya, it is customary to hire servants to help with household chores because there are no machines, and hiring housekeepers helps with job growth and the local economy.

You'd think you are in little India as you entered Macupa Flats, which is the gated community/complex I lived in. The smell of Indian spices, curries, chapattis, and basmati rice wafted from each house, making your mouth water, but the ramblings between the lady of the house and the servants brought you back to reality. "*Fagia nyumba, osha viombo na nguo.* (Sweep the floors, wash the dishes and clothes)."

Each household had at least one servant whose monthly pay averaged 5000 Kenyan Shillings (US$50). Every morning, the gates opened up, and they marched down to their respective employer's house an hour after sunrise, leaving their own children and family so they could look after someone else's. Before the sun's intense heat and humidity reached this corner of Kenya, most servants completed laundry (which was usually done outdoors and included clothes and school uniforms) from the day before that were drenched in sweat. *Thump, swish, thump, swish, scrub, scrub, thump, swish* could be heard from every household in the mid-morning as the servant scrubbed the clothes, slapped the piece of clothing on the cement pad to remove excess water, wrung the garments out, and then flapped them around before hanging them to dry on a clothes line.

Between noon and 2 pm, the sun scorches this part of the earth. It's too hot to even touch the steering wheel of a car or step barefoot on the road. During this time, the servants worked indoors as they dusted, mopped the floor, and ironed clothes for the next day. As the clock chimed 5:00 pm, the mosquito nets were set over the beds and dinner preparations were completed. Then they marched back out of the gates into their personal world.

We had two servants, Janet and Isaac, who were around until my pre-teenage years. Janet, a short and stout Kenyan woman, couldn't read or write, but she was like a second mother. She fed us when we were hungry and cleaned up after us. She died of AIDS, and we heard of many more servants dying of this disease as it became rampant in Kenya and in other parts of Africa. Then came Halima, a Muslim nanny. She always smiled and covered her hair with a bandana, and I felt I could talk to her about anything. "You can't speak Kiswahili, or you have problem speaking?" Halima asked in Kiswahili one day.

"I can speak K-k-iswahili, but I have difficulty speaking," I replied embarrassingly, thinking that now even the servants thought I was weird.

"You were born like this?" she asked curiously.

"I don't know, it's just the way I am. People make fun of me," I answered in Kiswahili and stuttered at the same time.

"What do they say?"

"They just mock me, but that doesn't bother me. It's the way people look at me. That bothers me. They look at me like I'm stupid or something."

"I don't think there's anything wrong with you. Some people are born mute and at least you have a voice. You are smart and have a good brain. Remember, no one can take that away from you," she said as she continued to chop onions and tomatoes for our next meal.

Halima is still with my mom, and she has been for over 30 years. When servants stay with a family for a long time, they become an extension of that family.

During school holidays, my mother let the servants take their annual leave of absence and she gave us a list of chores to complete. This began during one summer holiday. All of the kids sat around the house and fought most of the time or played outside all morning and evening and bossed the servants around. I think it was my mother's way of teaching us a lesson when she gave Janet and Isaac a leave of absence for two weeks and handed each one of us a list of chores to complete.

"Oh Mummy, please don't do this. It's our holiday," pleaded one of my siblings.

"I'm sorry, Janet and Isaac need a holiday, too, and I have to go to work. So someone has to do the chores around here. For each chore you do, I'll give you five cents each, and you'll notice how fast that adds up within two weeks."

"Can we spend the money on anything we want?" one of us asked.

"Yes, you can spend it on chocolate, soda, snacks, whatever you want. Or you can save it," she replied.

At the end of the day when mom came home, we all rushed up to her to show off what we had accomplished from dusting to cutting vegetables to ironing clothes and even making chappatis (tortillas) from scratch. This continued every year until I graduated from chores to working in the bakery at the age of twelve.

My mother was a busy woman and even though she could send one of the servants to the market, she'd take my sister and me to the town market to purchase fruits and vegetables for the week. She believed she could strike a better deal than her household help could.

Every Saturday as I entered the market, the smell of rotten vegetables and human sweat hit me instantly, and I automatically used my thumb and finger to plug my nose. As we walked around, vendors yelled to get my mother's attention. "Mama, tomato *bei nzuri* (I will give you a good price for tomatoes)." "Mama, pineapple *yote zimeuziwa, baki mbilitu. Nunua basi* (All the pineapples today have been sold; I'm only left with two. Better buy them now)." As my sister and I carried a sisal basket, we watched my mother negotiate with the vendors. "Tomato *nzuri lakini bei gali. Nitanunua mbele* (Your tomatoes are nice, but too expensive. I'll buy it from someone else up front)," mom replied, and instantly, the vendor would drop his price.

The market floor was filthy with fruit peels and mashed vegetables, and trying to side-step each was a challenge. The smell of sweat disappeared to be replaced with the smell of sweet mangoes and citrus fruits. I recall a time when one of the vendors sliced a ripe mango in front of me and offered a slice each to me and my sister. Biting into the succulent mango made the moment standstill; everyone and everything was quiet—it was just me and the sweet, heavenly taste of mango in my mouth. I looked back at the vendor, hoping he would give me another piece, but instead he said, *"Mzuri? Sema mama unataka kununua* (Nice? Tell your mother you want her to buy this)." I looked at him, smiled and replied, *"Nipa bei mzuri, tanunua. Bei gali, tanunua kwamwenzako* (Give us a good price and we will buy. If expensive, we will buy from your friend down the road)."

I guess going to the market wasn't a bad idea after all. I was learning the art of negotiating! After a while, the crowd, the smell, the noise of vendors yelling and buyers negotiating, and the sounds of live chickens clucking became overwhelming, and one could not wait to step outside onto the street and take a breath of fresh air.

My sister and I would carry the sisal basket to the car and beg my mother to go home so we could play with our friends. "You want to go to the beach tomorrow?" Mom would ask.

"Yes, yes, pleeeeease!" we'd yell.

"We have to do this first, then you have to finish your homework, okay?"

"Okay," we chorused because we knew the beach was more fun than playing with friends on Saturday afternoon, and again, this was a reward for helping at the market.

Our favourite day of the week was Sunday, which we always looked forward to because that day was spent at the beach. Mom and her sisters would prepare East Indian snacks like *samosas* (fried pastries), *bhajias* (potato and onion fritters), *karikababs* (fried meatballs), and all this had to be accompanied with masala chai tea in a thermos. As we drove to the beach, my mother and one of her sisters would talk about their businesses, challenges, and personal problems, and it was intriguing for me to know my mother from a different angle and to understand her trials and tribulations.

"Guli, there's a shortage of flour in the market. How are you coping with the bakery production?" Auntie Nurjehan, who had the same business as my mother, asked.

"Yes, the price of flour has increased, too, and it's really affecting our profit margin. It's such a hassle to call the flour mills everyday begging for more flour, but even they are in a bind and can't fulfill our orders. How can we meet the demands of our consumers? We can't even increase the price of bread because of government restrictions!" Mom said with exasperation.

"I hope this shortage ends soon. Guli, I want your opinion about one of my children? You know…" and so the conversation continued.

As we drove to the beach, the sisters would counsel each other on how to handle situations with children or the recent argument each had with her husband, and it seemed that this "Sunday car therapy" was what they looked forward to because they laughed, they cried, and they knew they were always there for each other, no matter what. These conversations about changes, obstacles, and conflict equipped me with coping mechanisms and taught me that life is like a slinky: it can stretch, it can twist, it can be uncomfortable, but in the end with real support, there's always hope and one can bounce back.

Even though there were rewards for completing chores and going to the market, I learned about responsibility, work ethic, and the idea of fulfilment. Creating responsibility is not just about giving someone a task to do. Responsibility is based on two aspects: accountability and empowerment. I was held accountable with a list of things to complete, and if they weren't done, then I'd be rewarded less. In addition, by giving me a list, my mother installed in me that there would be NO excuses or blame game for work that was not completed.

Creating excuses or blaming others for uncompleted work creates a victim mentality, which doesn't solve problems. Most of us create excuses and procrastinate or blame the busyness in our life for not getting something done. In essence, what we are doing is playing the victim role. When we blame something or someone else in our life, we are actually sending a message to our subconscious that says, "I'm a victim of that thing or label." On the other hand, my mother empowered me with decision-making on how the chores got done on my own terms, and this created the belief of capability and maturity.

Work ethic came from watching my parents work at their business. They started their day at 4 am in order to get breakfast on the table for us and to get to the bakery nice and early. By the time we came home for lunch, mom had lunch prepared for us, and we'd eat as a family. Right after lunch, we'd head back to school while mom and dad took a one-hour nap before heading back to the bakery to collect the sales of the day and to prepare the production for the next day. In the evening, we helped each other with homework while mom and dad looked at spreadsheets and accounts for the day and answered calls from drivers who hadn't made it back to the bakery because the truck had broken down. Moreover, doing the chores that the servants usually did made us more compassionate toward them because only then did we realize how hard they worked. But what made it even more significant was when I learned how far the servants had to travel to come to our place. Janet would walk for half an hour to the bus stop and then take the bus to our house, which could take another half an hour to an hour, depending on the number of stops it made.

These experiences taught us to prioritize, be responsible, value time, make effort, and have passion, because in the end when you see the rewards of what you've done, you feel fulfilled. One of the strengths of resilient people is their habit of setting an INTENTION. Intent comes from the Latin word *intendo*, which means to "stretch forward." My parents always said, "As long as you have your mental capacity, your hands and your legs, you can go for what you want and never live off of anyone." This statement alone created a victor mentality.

When you set the intention for what you want, you're already telling the universe that *it is possible*. You can go from intent to fulfilment by asking the following questions:

1. What's my intent?
2. Why is it important to me? This question sets the value you are placing on your purpose or goal.

3. What am I willing to do to get what I want? This question sets you up for being responsible and accountable.

4. What am I willing to give up to get what I want? This question makes you "stretch forward" and create the grit or mental toughness to keep you motivated. Note: You want to take pleasure in what you do so you can feel fulfilled.

5. What is stopping me now? This question makes you aware if you're lacking resources or creating procrastination because of your fears.

6. What are my strengths and how can I use them?

7. What resources do I need and how can I get them? This question gets your wheels turning.

8. How will getting what I want make me feel fulfilled? This question enables one to create a measurement of fulfilment by citing evidence.

Chapter 5

Fear

When I skipped grade 1 and started grade 2, I was scared, but knowing that I had friends, my older siblings, and their friends around me was comforting. I remember an office manager leading me to my classroom on that first day, and as I stepped into the room, I saw the teacher and gulped. "She looks *kali*!" I thought to myself. *Kali* in Kiswahili means "strict." She wore a simple cotton dress with print that gathered around her skinny waist, and she held a stick in her hand. "Welcome. You can sit there," she said in her thick Kenyan accent and pointed at a desk with her stick. As I searched to where she was pointing, I noticed a sea of faces staring at me and smiling. I didn't smile back. I walked to my desk to sit down.

There were about thirty wooden desks in the room—the kind that had a lid—and these desks were paired to form a row going down the classroom. Seated at those desks were a mixture of students from various backgrounds. It was a sea of black and brown faces: native Kenyans, East Indians, and Arabs, all in green and white uniforms.

"Can you tell us your name?" the teacher asked.

"Z-z-z-aheen." I stuttered and looked away, but I saw the look she had on her face. It was one of concern and surprise.

"Do you have your textbooks?" she asked again. I nodded up and down. "Okay class, take out your English reading book, and we are going to read the first story. You are each going to try and read a full sentence. Let's start at the front of the class and go down this line." I removed the reading book from my backpack and opened it to follow along. As each student read a sentence, I thought, *They read nicely*. My heart started thumping faster, and I clenched my hands together tightly, hoping that would calm me down or stop my heart from beating so hard. Then, it was my turn. I heard the teacher say, "Zaheen, read your sentence."

I saw my words clearly, and I opened my mouth to read aloud, "The c-c-c-cat a-a-a-and...." As I tried to read the sentence as fast as I could, I thought, "The teacher is getting mad. Is she going to spank me?" As I came to the end of the sentence, I sighed with relief as my classmate picked up the next sentence, but I snuck a look at my teacher, and she was staring at me with her mouth half open and then she looked back at her book.

In the days and months to follow, sentences became paragraphs, and it became more difficult for me to read.

"Zaheen, can you see me after class?" the teacher asked one day.

"Yes, teacher." I went up to her after the bell rang.

"You have trouble speaking?" she asked, and I nodded. "It's called stammering," she continued. "If it's a sentence, you can read, and if it's a long paragraph, I may let you skip. Do you understand?" I nodded and walked back to my desk feeling relieved that I didn't have to feel like a freak in front of my classmates or get teased for stuttering.

Reciting prayers aloud in a congregation at the age of eight is part of our culture, and I remember wearing a new dress that my mother had made by a local seamstress. It was a yellow cotton dress with pink polka dots and short, puffy sleeves. The dress had pretty pink lace that bordered the sleeves and the bottom of the dress, which reached my knees.

It was now my turn to sit on the stage, and I was shaking and nervous. The microphone seemed alive and scary, like it was about to zap me. I took a deep breath to calm myself down and kept wringing my hands so the shaking might stop. I heard the signal to begin and opened my mouth to recite, but nothing came out. I let out a sound from my vocal cords, but the sound was stuck at the top of my throat; I tried desperately to push out the word, and finally I spit it out as if a cork had been dislodged from my vocal cords. After a few words of recitation it happened again, but then it was different. "A-a-a-a-alha." I sounded like a scratched record. This kept happening and I was scared. *I want to finish now, help!* The recitation that was supposed to take 10 minutes, took 20. I thought it'd never end.

When a child says the prayer for the first time, he or she is rewarded with money from immediate and extended family members. As my aunts and uncles came up to me after all prayers were completed, none of them genuinely told me I did a good job. As they handed me money, I heard, "Did you practice enough?" "Next time practice more, okay?" "That is a nice dress you wore today." In each and everyone's eyes, I saw the look of embarrassment, the look of avoiding the subject, and even when they did say I did a good job, they had the look in their eyes that said, "There is something wrong with you."

As I started becoming aware of my speech and these hidden meanings behind people's perceptions of me, I formed my own meanings and mental frames that guided my behaviour:

"No one will like me if I stutter."

"I have to stop speaking like this, but the more I try, the worst it gets."

"I will just keep quiet in situations where I don't want to draw attention."

"I am so ashamed."

"I have to do better. I can't let them down."

In time, the teachers at school, my friends at school, and the people in Macupa Flats, as well as other people around me, got used to the way I spoke. My coping mechanisms included avoiding speaking to groups of three or more, saying no to anything that involved public speaking, and getting others to do the talking for me. At the same time, I devoured books so I could lose myself in another world and learn words and synonyms that I could substitute for words that started with a consonant that I found difficult to say like, T, K, S, C, P, B. Avoidance and complacency became my best friends, and people around me enabled my avoidance behaviour because they felt sorry for me; my environment remained the same, so complacency set in until I arrived in Alberta, Canada.

Attending school in Edmonton, Alberta, I continued to avoid speaking. I even told my teacher that I didn't want to read aloud or partake in presentations because I stammered. I met with a speech therapist while attending school, and she gave me some breathing techniques and asked me to slow down when I spoke, but a part of me refused to practice because I sounded even more freaky and weird when I talked really slow or elongated my consonants. I did it with her so that she would get off my back, and after a few sessions, she said, "Zaheen, it seems you've progressed quite well, and your stutter is not very severe. With practice, you'll do fine."

What a relief that was to hear. I really enjoyed grade 9 because I started making my own friends instead of hanging out with my sister's friends. I felt accepted, and I really enjoyed the school system in Canada. The teachers were so encouraging, there was no corporal punishment and no parents around to tell you what to do, and the neighbours that didn't care what you did. Back in Macupa Flats, no one could get away with anything and rumors literally spread like fire.

I didn't want to be different. I just wanted to fit in with my teenage friends, be normal, and have fun.

I started to use my old tricks of using synonyms that didn't have a consonant I couldn't say, or I'd pretend I had a sore throat on the day I had to present in class, or I'd beg my classmates to take care of public speaking while I completed the research part of a group project. Outside of school, my sister did most of the talking for me when it came to answering the phone, calling a business, going to the bank, paying bills, ordering a pizza, or even going shopping. These were all methods that I had incorporated into my life to cope better, but in reality, these behaviours were only doing one thing: making me the queen of avoidance. I thought I was being really smart by hiding my stutter and masking the real me, but in essence, I was allowing my stutter and my fears of stuttering to hold me prisoner.

Unfortunately, fears get the best of a person because we view fear as a demon that holds us captive and has control over us. However, we forget that fear is only an emotion, and it's our emotions that empower us or weaken us. Instead of ignoring, giving in, or numbing your fear, find the hidden meaning or positive intention behind your fear and acknowledge that. The hidden meanings behind my fear of stuttering were centered on these things:

- being different
- coming across as dumb (stereotype)
- getting teased
- being isolated by my friends

As I came to understand what my fears were centered around, I realized that my fear was keeping me safe from being embarrassed, and that I had taken up coping mechanisms. However, hiding behind those coping mechanisms and masking the real me caught up to me in the end.

What internal fears do you have? Do you fear public speaking, starting your own business, or changing your career? Do you fear failure or something entirely different? List three things that are keeping you from doing what you love because of your fear, and for each one ask, "How is fear helping me here in a positive way?" As you become aware of the hidden meaning behind your fear, acknowledge it instead of ignoring it.

Chapter 6

Embracing Fear

I attended the University of Alberta and received my bachelor's degree in food science and nutrition, but it was during this time that I had to face my fears, acknowledge my avoidance behaviours, and deal with the chaos within me.

In one of my classes, an assigned project involved partnering up with a colleague and inventing a food product and its benefits in the marketplace. I went into panic mode; my heart started beating, and my hands broke into a cold sweat. I thought of my usual avoidance mechanism: "I'll talk to my colleague and my professor. I'll do most of the work, but my colleague can present it all."

"Sir, I can't do the presentation you've asked," I said softly in the professor's office.

"Why not? You've been doing really well in this class," he asked surprised.

"What I mean is I'll do the work, but I'm going to get my partner to present it all. Is that going to affect my grade?" I asked with hesitation, but he still looked at me confused. "Sir, I stutter, and I won't be able to speak in front of the whole class," I explained.

55

"You stutter? I don't hear you stuttering right now," he said incredulously.

"I hide it really well, and I feel comfortable with you," I replied meekly.

"Zaheen, I'm sorry, but you have to present it, and if you don't, it will affect your grade."

"Sir, please understand I can't; I beg you. I can present it to you in your office, but not in front of the class, please," I pleaded.

"I'm sorry, that's not how I grade my students, and that's final," he replied firmly, indicating the conversation was over, but I could see the emotions playing out in his face. He felt sorry for me, and yet he wanted to grade the entire class fairly.

As I rode home on the public transit bus, I stared out the window feeling helpless and hopeless. I panicked all the way home. *I've come so far trying to get away from public speaking and presenting; surely I can't fail now!* I imagined myself standing in front of the class and trying to explain our project, and the images I held in my head were of me not getting the words out, as though they were stuck at the top of my throat, and my face contorting to spit the words out, all while seeing the expression of pity, surprise, and suppressed laughter on the faces of my fellow classmates. These images and thoughts I was having made me want to dig a hole and bury myself in it. *This can't be it! There has to be someone that can help me!*

I remembered confiding to one of my cousins about my speech impediment, and she had told me to visit the speech therapy department at the university, but I had dismissed it. My stop arrived. I got off the bus and rushed home to find the phone book (which we used a lot back then) and I frantically looked under SPEECH. As I trailed my finger down the page, I came across only one name: Institute of Stuttering Treatment and Research, also known as ISTAR. I looked up at the clock. *Hmm, it's only 3:30 pm; they might be open. Should I phone them or go there tomorrow?* I looked back down at the page to find an address, but I didn't see one. I stared at the touch-tone phone, wanting desperately to pick up the receiver and dial the number. *Oh, what's the worst thing that will happen—you'll stutter! That's what they hear all the time, so big deal!* I picked up the receiver and dialed the number.

"Thank you for calling ISTAR," a gentle voice answered.

"He-e-llo, my n-name is Z-zaheen," I said.

"Yes, how can I help you?" The person deliberately slowed down her rate of speech.

"I want to see someone. I stutter," I said quickly with a sigh of relief.

ISTAR was on the university campus, and after my first consultation, I was told I was a covert stutterer. This meant that I had built coping mechanisms to hide my stutter, but they were not serving me. Instead of dealing with my speech impediment, I was masking it the wrong way. I couldn't afford the cost of a three-week speech therapy intensive program, but the Elks Foundation of Canada came to my rescue and offered to pay the tuition fee. I'm eternally grateful for organizations like the Elks of Canada who make it their mandate to support a cause like improving speech and hearing impediments.

In three weeks, I learned how to slow down my rate of speech, I learned breathing techniques to allow me to speak easily, and I learned how to use the parts in my mouth to form and say words that were difficult for me. During the last week, I had to do things that I had always avoided: use the phone and make a speech. I'd always wanted to order pizza and have it delivered, but I could never do it because I couldn't say the words "pizza" and "delivery." On my last day, after a lot of practice and role playing on the phone, I ordered pizza at ISTAR and delivered my speech to a room full of strangers.

However, within three weeks of finishing at ISTAR, I was working at it on my own without any coaching or encouragement, and it was difficult. Here I was, looking for a cure to get rid of my stutter, and it was still there. Furthermore, my fear of speaking and my behavior of avoiding certain speaking situations came back to haunt me again. I was back at square one. *I thought this therapy would cure me, but it didn't work!*

I had a follow-up appointment with my speech therapist at ISTAR a few weeks later, and by then, I was prepared to tell her that the therapy didn't work for me. I walked up the stairs into the reception area and waited for my turn to see her.

"How are you doing Zaheen?" she asked with a slower rate of speech as we were in her office.

"Not good. I thought I wouldn't stutter anymore after the three-week program, but I still am, and I'm still avoiding speaking situations. I tried to use the phone to call for a pizza, and I just couldn't," I replied with a sigh of sadness.

"Have you been practicing the skills we taught you, and are you listening to the tape we gave you?" she asked. The cassette tape included follow-along practice sessions.

I shook my head from right to left and avoided eye contact.

"Zaheen, learning these skills and tools takes time and practice. It's not a cure. I want you to think back to the time you gave that speech and made your first pizza delivery call. Did you feel good?"

I nodded up and down and smiled.

"Yes, you did so well because you focused on the skills and practiced until you felt comfortable."

"But that was here. I felt comfortable, and I had help," I argued.

"This was a new environment for you, too, and it took you time to get comfortable, didn't it?" she stated assertively.

"I'm scared of sounding different, but I'm mostly scared of doing the things I've always avoided. I don't want to stutter anymore," I said desperately.

"I see, so your fear is holding you back from using the new resources we've given you," she said and stayed silent. I didn't say anything either. After a pregnant pause, she leaned forward in her chair and continued, "Zaheen, you have a choice and a decision to either stay where you are or use the resources we've given you and start practicing. Face your fear!"

As I walked out of ISTAR that afternoon in a daze, replaying the conversation in my head, I felt disappointed that I didn't get the answer I was looking for. But then suddenly, I heard a whisper, "Your fear is holding you hostage." I stopped walking, looked deeply into the green grass beneath me for what seemed like a long time and took in a deep breath. Something shifted in me because I looked up and said, "I'm not going to be held back by fear. I can do this." I started planning in my head how I could use the resources that I'd learned at ISTAR. I made a list of a few words I couldn't say and a list of simple things I had avoided before but that seemed within the realm of my capabilities.

I never liked wearing a watch, but I could never ask a stranger for the time either. One day, I went to the mall and started asking strangers for the time, and I kept doing that until I could say the word "time" subconsciously, without thinking about my breathing techniques or the tools I had used. It sounded funny at first when I'd take a breath before saying the word "time" and then softly releasing the "t" sound. Once I felt confident that I could execute this without avoiding it, I went to the next thing on my list and conquered that.

When a person decides to do something, he or she is either fully committed or not. Full commitment comes from being 100 percent responsible for any slip-ups, decisions, or actions. What this means is that there can be no excuses or blame games. Commitment comes from knowing that you'll give it all it takes and there's no going back. You have to be ready and want it more than anything else, and in the process, you'll learn more about yourself, your strengths, and your weaknesses.

I learned that I had allowed the shackles of fear to hold me in my comfort zone, and it had a positive intention—to keep me safe. But, I wasn't going anywhere. I was stuck in the same place year after year and feeling miserable about myself and my life. I kept on hating myself and feeling worthless. It's interesting that most of us feel this way, yet we remain in this comfort zone and still do nothing. This is madness.

The first catalyst that helped me slowly undo the shackles of fear was my professor. At first, I was angry at him for not being more understanding. But I realized that I was playing the victim again. *Oh, feel sorry for me!* By refusing my request, he indirectly sent a message that I needed to stop avoiding my problem. He knew that it would catch up to me later, and he was also preparing me for the real world where I had to make these kinds of presentations if I was to make it in my career.

The second catalyst in my journey was my speech therapist who saw through me and told me what I needed to hear. She could have told me to practice and come back after two weeks, but she didn't. What she did do really well was use the notion of "motivation by pain" to get me to take action. She made me realize that if I were to use the same default mechanisms I had used over the last 15 years, and continue in that same way, I'd feel more frustrated with myself. Imagining this caused me pain, and I didn't like being in pain. In fact, human beings don't like feeling pain and discomfort, and this feeling motivates us to take action. In addition, she also suggested moving toward a goal. This is "motivation by reward," where if I were to practice the resources and skills I'd been given, I'd be able to do the things that I was able to do on the last day of the program, which was to order pizza for delivery and be comfortable with public speaking. That feeling of achievement was beyond any feeling I'd ever had.

I'm not sure if she was aware that she had used classic human behaviour psychology to help me shed the disguises that had helped me stay captive in my own prison.

Many people are shocked when I tell them I stuttered and was not able to do the things that I can today. "But you speak so well, and you are so articulate," they say. If they only knew the truth of how much effort it took to change my mindset and behaviours. My "a-ha" moment occurred when I walked out of ISTAR and heard that whisper, but that was only the beginning of a long journey. There are times when I still stutter, and it can stay with me for a few weeks, and then there are times I won't even notice. The difference is, when I do stutter now, it doesn't have the emotional charge that it used to have. I think differently of myself because over time I have changed my belief system from *I'm not capable* to *I'm capable*. I've changed my mind set from *I can't speak and I don't have an opinion* to *I can speak, I want to speak, and I do have an opinion that counts.*

It took a long time to find my voice, and most successful people will agree that there is no magic pill or silver bullet to success. It takes time, effort, and consistency. When I had been doing the same thing for 15 years of my life, I couldn't have expected that things would change overnight, mainly due to the belief systems I had created. These belief systems guided my behaviour in a certain way. However, when I made the decision to embrace fear, I also made the decision to practice my new-found resources and skills every day. Every morning as I'd get ready to go to university, I'd play the cassette tape and follow along with the practice session to make my speech smoother. I used this same formula of practice and replacing old habits with new and improved habits when I changed my relationship with food.

Praying out loud was always a contentious issue because it took me back to the time I was eight years old. But I practiced at home and said my prayers out aloud, using my new speech skills, even though no one was there to hear me. It was only after I got married at 25 years old that I took the plunge to say prayers aloud. The experience was excruciating but at the same time, I said to myself, *You can do it.*

Between the ages of 19 and 25, I had only accomplished a few of the things on my list that I had avoided, such as ordering food, asking for directions, and even working at a grocery till. I still hadn't tackled the phone completely, and I still shied away from public speaking. Interestingly, I also realized that it was only in my late thirties that I got comfortable with voicing my opinion at meetings; I had never done that before.

Notice the two Cs I keep mentioning in this chapter: Commitment and Consistency. Commitment occurs when one has decided wholeheartedly, without a shadow of a doubt, to create a life change, face obstacles, and find a way to overcome barriers. Consistency occurs when one decides to create a daily, weekly, or monthly practice that will help along the journey. Without consistency, commitment can become lost, and without commitment, consistency doesn't follow through. A car cannot be driven unless there's gas, but even if there is gas, it doesn't necessarily mean that the car will be driven; it can sit in a garage and never be used.

What are you willing to commit to in order to take your life or business to the next level? What consistent actions are you willing to implement to move forward in life or business?

Chapter 7

Entrepreneur

An entrepreneur is someone who sees an opportunity, makes a plan, and executes the business knowing there are risks involved. I don't think one is born an entrepreneur, and it's certainly not in one's DNA; however, a person becomes an entrepreneur if he or she has a purpose, wants to tap into some unique creativity, or is exposed to it from a young age.

When I tell people that I moved from Kenya to Canada, their first reaction is usually to say, "But you don't look African, so how's that possible?" I explain how during the colonial times, South Asians from British India were brought into East Africa to help build the railway line because they already had experience building rail in India. Overtime, South Asians saw an opportunity to create trade routes, set up shops, and make East Africa their home. Therefore, every generation of African-Asians after that knew how to do business because they were born into it. They were natural entrepreneurs.

When the president of Uganda, Idi Amin, expelled all the South Asians in 1972, most of them had little education, but most had made their money in business. As they emigrated to the UK and to North America, some spoke little English and worked as labourers, hotel housekeepers, and janitors but after a few years, they saved up money to invest in businesses. My husband's parents came to Canada the same way and worked two jobs at $2 per hour while raising their children. After a few years, they invested in a German bakery which led them to become mortgage-free more quickly than expected. Now when I look back at this community of East Indians who had similar stories and sacrifices, I wonder if resilient traits or the practice of resilience is somehow passed subconsciously from one generation to another. Being entrepreneurs and leaders probably comes naturally to both my husband and me because we are both fourth-generation African-Asian and we've grown up watching businesses flourish or fail or be taken away by political instability. However, we've seen in our parents the drive to bounce back and start again as though it's normal. We've seen them go through changes in their life and use those changes as an opportunity to turn that challenge to their advantage. We've seen them remain committed to a sense of purpose—feeding and educating their families—to create stability. We've seen them remain in control of their emotions so that they can seek quick solutions instead of being stuck in overwhelm and worry. We've seen them have faith in a higher being because that gives them strength and hope. These traits have been modeled from one generation to another, but this also proves that modeling can be a strategy to success.

One of the presuppositions in neuro linguistic programming (NLP) is, *Possible in the world, possible for me.* Any skill, talent, or ability that an individual has can be broken down into its components and taught to anyone who does not have severe physiological or neurological damage. This is the basis of modeling and it has been proven in multiple cases. For example, when Roger Bannister managed to run a mile in four minutes, others followed suit.

One of those role models is my mother. She's always had a passion for creating new food products, and her drive has been to provide for the family while fuelling her passion. In the 1970s and 80s, there were few women entrepreneurs in Kenya, especially in the East Indian culture. Most women stayed at home or worked as administrative assistants in schools, hospitals, or offices. Our parent's lives revolved around the bakery, and this came home with them, too. After evening prayers and homework, except for my younger brothers, my older siblings and I would go into my parent's room and start counting coins from the day's sales. The coins were spread over the bed on a bed sheet, and we' be given the task to count one type of coin, either 25 cents or a shilling. I remember thinking then after seeing so much money on the bed night after night that *having a business makes me rich!*

Mom had a desire to make us entrepreneurs and leaders from a young age when it came to the bakery business. She even taught my sister and me how to drive a car. Once I hit the age of 12, we graduated from doing house chores during school holidays to working at the bakery. Our day started at 4:30 am with a visit to *jamatkhana,* where we meditated and prayed, and then we headed out to the lighthouse area where we walked for 20 minutes, breathing fresh air as the waves of the Indian Ocean crashed against the rocks, and the sun slowly peeked out of the pink and dark blue skies while the world slowly started to wake up.

One may wonder what on earth would make pre-teens want to wake up at 4:30 am. Surely, it wasn't the smell of fresh air! No, it was the excitement of learning how to drive. After the walk, mom would teach my sister and me to drive, and then we'd head to get some breakfast for the family, get ready, and go to the bakery.

On my first day, mom gave the floor supervisor some instructions then looked at me to say, "Zaheen, you are going to learn how we bake bread and what goes in it. You will listen to what the floor supervisor tells you because in two weeks, you will take over his position so he can go on holidays. Is that understood?" I nodded.

The floor supervisor looked at me and smiled, "*Toto ya mama* (child of madam), *taonesha bakery sasa hivi* (let me show you the bakery first)," he said in Kiswahili as he led me on while the smell of fresh baked bread filled the air.

He took me to the raw ingredients area and spoke in Kiswahili as he showed me how the raw ingredients—sugar, fat, yeast, and salt—were measured ahead of time for each 90kg bag of flour. He explained that this was the most important part of the production because it was the taste of these raw ingredients that made the bread. I nodded as I observed the workers measure and weigh each ingredient on a scale before placing them in a bucket. He then walked me to the mixing area where little buckets of raw ingredients sat near the big dough mixer. An African employee picked up the huge bag of flour and dumped its contents into the mixer before turning on the mixer blades. After a few seconds, he added the contents of one bucket that held the raw ingredients as well as some water and then waited for the dough to form.

Near the dough mixer was the kneading area where two workers were cutting a small amount of dough, weighing it on a scale, kneading it into an oval shape, and throwing them into loaf tins. I couldn't believe how fast they were, and I was hypnotized by the speed and continuous motion. "John, how many loaves of bread do you get from one bag of flour?" I asked the supervisor in Kiswahili.

"Three hundred and forty," he answered.

"How do you know how many loaves of bread to make for today?" I asked curiously. John smiled and explained that we have orders from businesses, and we also go by an average number from previous sales. We arrived at the second most important area, where the bread was proofed and baked. John pointed to the proofer and explained that bread has to rise to a certain level before it's baked in the ovens. I stared at the large deck ovens that were higher than even John, and as the baker opened one of the doors, the humid air became even hotter. The golden brown loaves of bread were removed from the ovens, and the smell made me want to take a loaf of bread, rip it open in the middle, and grab the soft whiteness and devour it. "Smells good, doesn't it?" John asked in Kiswahili as though reading my mind. I smiled.

"Here's the last stop in the production process," he explained as we arrived at slicing and packing. One person was weighing the baked bread to ensure it met food standards and then passed it on to the person in charge of two slicer machines that vibrated loudly. As the bread was sliced by a slicer machine, it was whisked up by the workers who placed it in a plastic bag, tied it up, and placed it in large square crates.

"What you saw is only the production system, which you have to understand because it is the foundation of all the other systems," John explained in Kiswahili. I looked at him in confusion and he explained further. "After the loaves of bread are packed, we have the loading system where each truck takes a certain amount to sell. This way we can then keep track of how many loaves of bread we made, how many were sold, and the sales we should make based on those numbers."

When John left on his holidays, Mom quizzed me on what I had learned—the amount of yeast, fat, sugar, flour, and the number of loaves that must come out from one bag of flour. And if we were to make a certain amount of loaves for the day, how many bags of flour would that be, and how many hours would that take, and so on. The next few weeks were exciting and challenging as I supervised adults, which increased my self-confidence, but also taught me a lot about being a leader. At 14 years old, I had graduated from floor supervisor to balancing the production and sales sheets. If these didn't balance, then there were holes in the system, and it was my job to find the leak.

These experiences not only taught me how to be an entrepreneur, but they taught me about the value of systems and organizing when building a business or a company. Just like our bodies have certain systems for different functions, for example, digestion, breathing, and immune, a company or business works better when there are systems in place. The whole business is the sum of its parts, and a business with inefficient systems leads to chaos. Earlier in the chapter, I mentioned how the South Asian culture modeled resilient traits from one generation to another. I may not use the same systems as a bakery, but I model some aspects of it and model businesses that are similar to mine to help me grow my businesses.

With creating efficient systems comes the responsibility of being organized so that things run smoothly, and stability is created. Having systems also makes it easier to have emotional resilience in times of difficulty because one of those systems may have to merge or be tweaked to make things a little more efficient if you have to do more with less.

Here are four reasons you need efficient systems in business:

1. **Business resilience**. In challenging times, a system may have to merge, be upgraded, or made obsolete to make things run more efficiently. Therefore, understand how each system works and why it's

important in your business. What does this system allow you to do and have? If you had to cut costs, which system could cause less impact? What steps are involved in each system, and which ones could be delegated or outsourced to create efficiency?

2. **Stay ahead of the game**. Even though we can't see inside our bodies, our bodily systems are running without us knowing. However, we may not know if they are running efficiently until a symptom develops. In my behaviour weight loss book, I mention that those who are aware and educated on how bodily systems work, take extra effort to plan ahead, organize their meals, and look ahead for any barriers that will impact their health. Similarly, to maintain and grow your business, plan ahead and look out for any potential barriers that could affect you. Keep abreast of new technology in your industry or marketing ideas that your competition is having success with. Find better and cost-effective systems to attract new clients, but connect with the clients you already have to remind them that you're still around.

3. **Be the CEO**. Some entrepreneurs and business owners feel like they have to do it all. I was there too,

and I realized I'd never grow to where I want to be because I'd still be "doing" rather than envisioning and fueling my passion. With the rise of the internet, outsourcing tasks through sites like Upwork and Fiverr has been phenomenal! As I was trying to run a household, work full time, operate a wellness centre, and re-brand and re-launch my speaking career, I decided that I couldn't keep "doing" because I'd always be catching up instead of leaping forward. I hired a local lady to clean my house every two weeks. I had to dig into my pockets, but I realized that the amount of time it freed up for me to concentrate on sending proposals, creating marketing campaigns, and spending extra time with my family was well worth it. I hired a virtual assistant through Upwork, and I asked my website designer to take on graphic design and social media planning to help me spread my message better.

4. **Consistent action**. This is the cornerstone of any successful business. Do you have a consistent marketing strategy? Do you consistently track growth? Do you consistently create? I created a system to plan my marketing:

a) Blog every week.

b) Google Hangout show every first and last Sunday of the month, and convert to podcast.

c) Send inquiry emails to podcast producers and conference chairs once a week with a follow-up.

d) Write a chapter for my book every Sunday.

e) Host a webinar six times a year.

f) Create two to three products a year, such as an audio series, online courses, or e-books.

In order to leap forward, you have to stop doing tasks that others can do easily with some instruction and take on an approach of being a CEO of your business and behave in that manner. Once you create systems and make it a habit, you will realize how less stressed you feel and how much more productive you are in fueling your passion and seeing greater returns.

With the operations of the wellness centre, we have similar systems and most are delegated to our receptionist and accountant, but at the end of the month, I spend time looking at all the systems from percentage of services offered, to the returns of a marketing campaign for the month, to customer relations.

To make a system work, you also have to be organized and build efficient habits. My parents started out baking bread, but soon enough it was delegated to people who could easily do it so they could generate ideas of finding new markets or developing new products. Similarly, I have found people who could do for me the small things in which I have no interest and which take away time from doing things I love. Everyone has mentors who are successful in a business similar to yours. Model after him or her and learn his or her habits, decision criteria, and belief systems and values. These beliefs and values are what guide your mentor's habits and behaviours, and the beliefs and values of my South Asian-African culture, passed from one generation to another, have helped me to get where I am.

Chapter 8

My Role Model

One of my role models is my mother, and I've always seen her carry herself with confidence even though she struggles with her weight. I believe it's because she puts more importance in her self-worth than her weight, and she doesn't let her weight get her down. She's been through many challenges, both personally and in business, and she seems to have always come through. My mother is a resilient person in the truest sense because she's always done what she's passionate about, she's been optimistic, she embraces change, she's a master at problem solving, and she handles her setbacks well.

My mother is assertive, but she also taught me the true meaning behind empathy and compassion, which is stepping into the other person's perspective. She raised six kids but only had four of her own, and I did not know any better until I was eight years old.

"Did you know Ashif and Nilu are not your real brother and sister?" one my friends blurted out while we played a board game.

"Of course they are," my sister Zohreen and I both replied.

79

"My mummy said that your daddy was married to someone else first," the friend continued.

My sister and I looked at each other with confusion then confronted my mother that same day while no one was listening. She sighed and nodded, "Yes it's true, I didn't give birth to them. Daddy was married before, and he had Ashif and Nilu with her." My sister and I were shocked! *Daddy was married before, and Mummy is his second wife and not his only wife? How is that possible?* I had all these thoughts going through my head: *Can we marry twice? Where is the first wife? Doesn't she miss her children? Why haven't we seen her?*

"How come you didn't tell us before?" Zohreen asked.

"I didn't want you treating them differently, and I want you to continue treating them just like you have been doing, like nothing has changed."

Step-mothers like my mother were rare at that time. She was right—she treated them like her own and never made any of us aware that they were not. She treated the servants in the house as well as the workers in the bakery with empathy when it was called for. Being a CEO or leader doesn't mean that one always has to be assertive and not show a compassionate side. In fact, that is what makes us human, and it allows us to lead better when we can step into another person's perspective.

I've witnessed and spoken to people who work for my mother and have been with her for a long time. They all say the same things about her: she's fair, she treats people with respect, she's positive, and she empowers employees by trusting them, she listens and she makes them feel important. Wouldn't you want employees in your organization talking about managers and leaders this way?

Her entrepreneurship skills came into play at a very young age because she had a purpose and saw an opportunity. At one point during her childhood, her purpose was to eat the expensive store candy, but she didn't have money and never got any from her father. Mom and her sisters settled with making home made candy called *Gudi*. She began sharing it with her friends, and they wanted more!

Mom's purpose was re-ignited, and she saw an opportunity: to sell her new product to her friends at a mere penny each. Business started picking up, and her sisters started helping her sell, but that didn't last long because all their profits were going into buying store-bought candy for themselves, and my grandmother found out and put an end to it.

It's interesting how experiences in our childhood carry on into our adult lives. Mom and her sisters have a sweet tooth even today. Moreover, Mom has always believed that she's a good cook (which she is), and she's always been interested in making new recipes for home meals or new products for the bakery. Growing up, she developed a knack for making cakes that were devoured quickly, and she thought nothing of it until one day, when still newly married, she gave some leftover cakes to dad's friends who convinced her to reformulate the product, keeping her ingredient cost down, so that she could market her cakes as snacks to local Kenyan workers.

During that time in Kenya, workers liked to spend the least amount of money to fill up their stomachs because every penny saved counted toward their children's health and education. Keeping the cost in mind while still making a good product was a challenge, but after several reformulations and taste-tests, she nailed it. Mom baked while Dad sold cakes to local shopkeepers who ordered more and more. After a few months, they had to invest in another domestic oven and hire some help, but again in a few months, the space at home wasn't enough because cakes were now getting packaged in bedrooms. This was the start of their bakery business.

When Ashif and Nilu were older and had completed college, Mom handed over the reins of the bakery in Mombasa to them because she wanted to open another branch in Nairobi, the capital city of Kenya. Her sister, who ran a similar business, seemed to be doing well in Nairobi, so we packed up and moved there while Ashif and Nilu handled the bakery in Mombasa. Things did not go well and within the two years that we were there, we lost almost everything.

We didn't lose it to political instability or rebels as most would think would have happened in Nairobi; instead, it was a slow and painful loss through lack of proper management, poor contracts, stealing, and poor planning. First, Ashif and Nilu had conflicts while operating the bakery in Mombasa because each had their own management style, which created chaos across departments. There is no blame game here, but there is a lesson to be learned about management styles and dividing the work rather than doing it all, even in small businesses. My husband and I have our own departments in our wellness centre and we have a meeting each week to discuss pending business matters without stepping on each other's toes.

Second, my parents were tapping into a market that was already loyal to other bigger brands, and they had little chance of breaking into this market. This is the typical brand story of David vs. Goliath. Third, working with people in fast-paced Nairobi is different than working with people in Mombasa, a more-laid back city. Work ethic is different, the level of education is different, and finding loyal middle managers and sales managers became difficult.

My parents kept injecting their savings to keep running both bakeries, but the time came when they couldn't afford to buy beef or chicken, and eating meat became only a weekend treat.

"Why do we keep eating rice and lentil soup for dinner?" I remember asking my mother one afternoon after school.

She bluntly answered, "We can't afford it." I looked at her with confusion and that evening Mom and Dad explained to us that times were tough, and we would have to make do with what we were given. After a few months, we moved back to our home in Mombasa, but the bakery in Mombasa was sold while the one in Nairobi was closed; all the equipment was sold to pay off all the debt my parents owed.

My mother told me the story of how they had to start all over again; all she knew how to do was run a bakery, and she was so passionate about it that she urged my dad to snap out of his depression and start looking for a place to start a bakery. My father, on the other hand, was adamant that he did not want to get into a business that took his savings and cost him his reputation. He wanted to start another business in which neither of them had any experience. Mom explained to him that they had done really well before, and she had an idea of how to reduce costs even more and increase profits, but Dad wanted nothing to do with it.

Mom rented a warehouse just off Mombasa Island, and she was terrified because she was told not only by her husband but also by others that she was putting up a bakery in the wrong area. She adopted a couple of strategies to decrease expenses and increase cash flow. The first was to remove the use of trucks to deliver bread into various areas and replace those with carrier bicycles that could safely carry a moderate load of bread. This would not only eliminate gas and auto repair expenses, but bicycles are cheaper to purchase, and they can be easily repaired or replaced. The second was to offer a commission to the bicycle vendor for every loaf of bread he sold; this would motivate him to sell more bread and take the bread into different communities around the area. The third was to open a bakery outside city limits and make bread more readily available to the smaller communities so the customers need not travel into the city for such a basic necessity. These tweaks in her business decreased her costs tremendously and increased her profit margins so much so that Dad decided to join her again.

Life is full of curve balls and challenges. Sometimes we make choices that put us on a very difficult path, but instead of beating ourselves up for taking that path, we can choose to react differently and consider a better outcome. My mother could have been a wicked a step-mother, but she chose to react with compassion and didn't even tell us about it until we asked. She chose to treat her employees as a true leader instead of yelling at them and disempowering them. In fact, most of her old employees returned to her when she re-opened a bakery after returning from Nairobi.

My mother admitted she probably made a mistake opening another branch in Nairobi without proper planning and market research, but that experience taught her a few things: to view her mistake as "feedback" because she took the lesson from that experience and asked herself, "How can I make it work this time around?" She focused on the solutions rather than the problems. My parents did so well the second time that their competitors took on their business model!

When we focus on our failures, we dwell on the past and the problems we experienced, which in turn, drives the fear of failure even deeper. Successful people think of failure as feedback. Why? It has three purposes: First, it stops the fear of failure in its tracks; second, feedback allows one to analyze the lessons learned from past experience; and third, putting the lesson to positive use leads to the creation of new possibilities and outcome.

If you think you are faced with failure, find an opportunity of growth by asking:

1. What do I want?

2. What do I have?

3. What have I learned from this experience?

4. What can I do differently?

5. What will be the evidence of my success?

PART 2 – Eight Keys for Resiliency

Chapter 9

Emotional Resilience

It is your reaction to adversity, not the adversity itself that determines how life's story will develop.

– Dieter F. Uchtdorf

I help people build their resilience muscle so it becomes the first reflex when faced with an obstacle or when finding themselves with their back against the wall. The first step to building that resilience muscle is understanding how to become more emotionally resilient, able to move forward, and release oneself from that feeling of being stuck. Wouldn't you agree that emotions affect our whole system: mind and body? Whether it's feeling fear or anxiety or worry, you may also feel it in some part of the body, such as weakness in the legs or a gnawing in the pit of your stomach or a faster heart rate. It's perfectly fine to feel this way instead of resisting these feelings and symptoms. Resilient people also feel fear and anxiety, but they refuse to let those feelings dominate and keep them stuck. Instead, they use all of their primary senses to change their thinking and bounce forward.

In my research, I have found there are three steps to building emotional resilience (ER): sensory intelligence (SI), emotional intent (EI) and emotional management (EM)

ER = SI+EI+EM

Sensory Intelligence (SI)

Sensory awareness involves becoming aware and building on the other senses rather than just focusing on the feelings that are dragging you down. When you walk into someone's house during a festive season like Christmas, you notice the colors, smells, and maybe even sounds of festive songs playing in the background, and you draw conclusions about the hosts. When building your emotional resilience, you want to become *sensory intelligent* by noticing the images you're bringing up (visual cues) and the things you say to yourself (auditory cues). Notice what happens inside your head and body when I ask you to think of the last time you had an argument. What images, thoughts, sounds or even smells come up?

In neuro linguistic programming (NLP), I was taught to pay less attention to *what* we think and more attention to *how* we think about something. As I learned to become more *sensory intelligent* and pay attention to how I was thinking, I realized I could control how I think about a person or a situation.

Emotional Intent (EI)

Our so-called negative emotions have a *positive intent*. For example, if you've been asked to present at the next board meeting, you may start feeling anxious and even scared, but we hardly ever acknowledge the reason behind those emotions. The *positive intent* of these feelings is to keep you safe from embarrassment. Once you acknowledge the positive intent behind the emotion, you are one step closer to emotional resilience.

Emotional Management (EM)

When we drive into a parking lot, our intent is to park the car so we can go do what we came to do. Similarly, *emotional management* is like parking your emotions so you can focus on what you want rather than what you don't want. In NLP, we call it *disassociation* or *emotional flexibility*. This is where we subconsciously step back and look at the situation objectively rather than emotionally.

When I changed my attitude about my fear of speaking, I didn't realize than that I was incorporating these three steps to create emotional resilience. I became aware of the images and thoughts I'd say to myself to avoid speaking (SI), I understood the positive intent behind my fear of speaking, which was that I didn't want to be perceived as stupid when

I spoke (EI), and I parked my fear to one side. I took a step back and looked objectively at my situation. I realized that what I wanted was to speak well without the feeling of fear or doubt. With that objective in mind, I could see myself taking action and using the skills I had learned from ISTAR. Holding these new images in my head propelled positive feelings and guided my behavior to do the very thing I had avoided before (EM).

In 2012, my husband and I leased an expensive piece of equipment to complement the services we offer at the wellness centre. We did our homework by looking at the projections for the community we lived in, we spoke to other centres that had similar equipment, and we even spoke to our accountant. All encouraged us to get it, and guess what—we lost a lot of money. We had to inject our own savings in the beginning to make the monthly lease payments. I can recall a time when I was sitting at home having my tea, but my thoughts and self-talk were focused on a failing business: *What if we can't make the payment next month? I can't keep injecting money into this. Let's sell this business because this is too much. I should have listened to my strong gut feeling instead of listening to others.* These thoughts kept circulating. I suddenly became aware of the empty feeling in the pit of my stomach, which drew my attention to my self-talk, and I intentionally focused on the images I was holding. They were images of being bankrupt, losing the business, and even losing my home. I put my hand to my mouth and wanted to cry. *Why am I doing this to myself,* I thought. *Manage your emotions, Zaheen and find a way!* This is all *sensory intelligence* where I'm becoming aware of what I'm visualizing, feeling (kinesthetic) and saying to myself (auditory).

I focused on what I wanted instead of what I didn't want, and that was how we started making this service work and making money from it. As soon as I changed my words and acknowledged my anxiety, I started feeling better and noticed the images I held had disappeared. I then began to re-program my thinking by asking some critical questions.

I also used the practice of emotional resilience in my job as a public health inspector. With a job like mine, there can be stressors or challenges every day, but I'm sure other careers in health care or public service have the same challenges.

Whether you are facing a work conflict or challenge, use the first step, sensory intelligence, to become aware of the following:

- what you are seeing in your mind's eye (visual)
- your self-talk and/or thoughts or sounds (auditory)
- your feelings or bodily symptoms (kinesthetic)

If you think you've been placed in a difficult position or are working with a difficult situation, ask yourself, "What's the positive intent behind (this situation, this person's behaviour)?" Simultaneously, acknowledge any feelings you're having and know they are there for a reason.

Next, manage your emotions by stepping back or disassociating from your emotional self and looking at it objectively. At this stage ask, "What do I want?" and ensure the answers are stated in the positive not the negative.

When I was faced with difficult situations while working as a health inspector, I'd get anxious. However, not only did I step back and look objectively at the situation, which released the anxiety, I also stepped into the other person's perspective to understand what they're seeing in their mind's eye or feeling, and I often empathized with them. In fact, my supervisor often commented on how calm I was in a tense situation and how well I defused the conflict.

Someone once told me we think in pictures, and it's these pictures that guide our thoughts and behaviors. If I believe that I'm not going to succeed, then the images I hold in my head will be those of self-pity and struggle. My thoughts will follow the pattern and my behaviors will sabotage any success. Thinking in pictures is similar to watching TV in our head. However, when we watch TV, we tend to choose and control what we want to watch, and thanks to the remote control, we can change channels pretty quickly! When I'm flipping channels, and I come across a horror movie, I quickly change the channel because I don't like watching horror. Yet, we tend to refuse to do that very same thing in our head, where our mind's channel is mostly tuned to negative and catastrophic images.

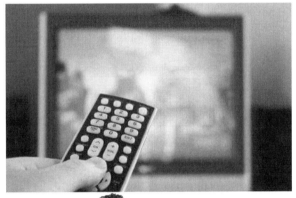

Resilience REFLEX   Unlock the Power of You

Start flipping those images in your head as though you are watching TV. Have an imaginary remote control where you can control the channel button for your images, the volume button for your self-talk, and you can even STOP or PAUSE what you are watching in your head to reflect, and then press START again. Here's a bonus: A person can even record the happy moments, positive images, or actionable steps taken to achieve success in one area and replay that to access some learning opportunities.

One of the founders of NLP, Richard Bandler, once said, "If I came over to your house and painted an ugly picture on your wall, you'd paint over it, yet people leave those ugly pictures in their minds year after year."

Here are some quick tools to keep in mind anytime you are faced with a challenge or conflict, or experience negative emotions like fear, worry, and anxiety. Remember, there's no magic wand; it takes practice:

- Notice your sensory cues: Visual, Auditory and Kinesthetic.

- Find the positive intent.

- Re-frame that negative feeling as a signal for finding a solution by asking, "What do I want?"

- Dissociate yourself and take a step back to view the situation objectively rather than emotionally. Think about parking your feelings like you'd park your car in a parking lot.

- Use an imaginary remote control to control the images you hold in your head.

Chapter 10

Reframe

Obstacles don't have to stop you. If you run into a wall, don't turn around and give up. Figure out how to climb it, go through it, or work around it.

— Michael Jordan

Life continually throws different curve balls. Some will be large and others small, but the large ones take us to new levels of personal growth. Look back on your life and recall some catastrophic challenges, personal or professional, where you thought to yourself, "I don't how I'm going to get through this!" But you did, and now when you look back, you probably wonder, "I don't how I did it, but I got through this," or "I'm so grateful that (name) helped me."

At the time, you were stuck in the worry because it was overwhelming. As you worry and get overwhelmed, you are hindered by thoughts and images in your head about all the things that could go wrong; then, most of us avoid looking at the problem because we think it will go away or somehow get solved on its own. This is what distinguishes resilient people from the normal population. Resilient individuals also

97

suffer from worry and become overwhelmed. They also feel fear, but they remind themselves that if they don't find a solution, it will come back to haunt them, so they force themselves to look at the problem and look for ways to overcome.

In the previous chapter, I talked about emotional resilience and how a resilient individual uses a process to manage his or her emotions. The next step is to reprogram yourself to look for solutions rather than to dwell in the worry.

As you read this, you may think it sounds simple, but I'm surprised by how many people keep worrying and remain stuck instead of looking for solutions. It is as though their brain is wired to stay in this worrisome state while they think the problem will just go away somehow. In this chapter, you will learn a methodology for moving from stuck to forward, from being worried to feeling relieved, and from being scared to feeling confident. Your problem-solving muscle is in atrophy right now, and it needs to be worked so that the next time you think your back is against the wall and you don't have a solution, you can use this simple process to bounce back. This process takes practice, and it is only with that practice that you will improve.

When we decided to open a wellness centre, we knew nothing about running this kind of business. All we knew was we wanted to offer a place of healing and transformation. Having projections and a business plan was what the bank wanted, but the bigger problem was operating this business with proper systems in place. How were we going to do this? I re-framed my question to, "I'm sure I'm not the first one who has thought of this business. Who has done this and is willing to mentor me?" I contacted a few business owners who would be willing to teach me the systems they used, and one agreed to mentor me. I implemented his advice, and the operations ran smoothly with a few hiccups here and there.

A year and a half later, after we opened, my husband and I bought a medical laser machine with the capability of doing three laser modalities. This wasn't an inexpensive machine; it was similar to buying a small piece of land in our town! Just like any smart small business owner, we conducted market research and compared sales projections of similar businesses in similar populations, and we spoke to our accountant. For the first two years, as I mentioned earlier, we had to make the payments for the machine from our own savings. We advertised locally, placed Facebook ads, offered a 50 percent discount on market-based prices in the first month to our subscriber list, all to get people in the door; still, we couldn't meet those projections, let alone pay for the machine. I was tired of seeing my savings deplete, and I was tired of borrowing.

I recall having a discussion with my husband that we couldn't continue paying for this machine, and I felt we had tried everything. I went as far as to tell him that we had failed. For one week, I had a nasty feeling in the pit of my stomach, battling images of the business closing and feeling miserable about it. At one point, though, when I became really aware, I stopped and applied my technique of emotional resilience. Then I went on to reframe my thinking by stating and asking, "I'm sure I'm not the only who has had this problem. Who can help me figure out how to increase revenue from this service we are offering?" At the time, we were only offering one of the medical laser modalities. I started studying other successful centres and service industries and found a way to make it easier for the customer to purchase medical laser services. I realized that the number one hindrance for our customers in purchasing medical laser service packages was the cost. I spent time trying to figure out how we could increase revenue, and yet make it affordable for our customers. We started offering interest-free payment plans and combining package treatments, and this increased our revenue by 50 percent in three months.

I learned about re-framing problems in NLP, and this process really gets a person to think differently. By stating to myself that, "I'm not the only one who has this problem. There must be others who have solved similar issues," I separated myself from the worry and subconsciously sent a message to my brain that I was instead hunting for a solution. This approach of re-framing can be used in any area of life or business, and it helps to make the problem easier to deal with because now I start looking at it objectively rather than thinking about it emotionally and dwelling in the worry. When my mother found a way to deliver bread with bicycles instead of trucks, she re-framed her thinking by asking a simple question, "How can I increase cash flow, decrease costs, and have enough capital to start another bakery?"

There are several ways to re-frame a problem—to change the context of an experience so that you can change its meaning and consider it from a different perspective. Here are four examples of re-framing

1. Back to the Future: What if you could step six months into the future and look back to now and ask yourself, "What did I do to overcome the problem?"

2. Mentor Magic: Pretend you are your mentor and step into your mentor's shoes and ask yourself, "What

would I do to overcome this problem?" Make sure you are seeing life through his/her eyes and listening through his/her ears.

3. Toolbox: What if you had all the information you needed to get a solution? What information would you use from your toolbox to change the circumstance you are in right now?

4. Superhero Magic: Everyone had a superhero growing up, and mine was Wonder Woman. I loved how she'd spin to go from being ordinary to being extraordinary! What if you could be your superhero, or better yet, what if you imagined slipping into that superhero costume (you may even have an old Halloween picture to remind you!)? What "magic" would you use to change something within your problem?

When something goes wrong in life or business, we tend to have a pity party. *Oh, why is this happening to me?* Then, we tend to drag this into other areas of our life. Of course, one is allowed to have a pity party, but keep it short and go press the RESET button so you can step out of it and start solving the problem.

Once you RESET yourself, re-frame the problem by using one of the ways mentioned above, and then apply your findings with some flexibility. When you find someone who you can model, contact that person and ask if you can pick his or her brain over coffee or lunch; make sure you take some action before contacting that person again.

The simple process of problem solving is:

1. Reset (applying emotional resilience)
2. Reframe
3. Apply flexibility

When you reset yourself using the emotional resilience method and then reframe, you will automatically start finding solutions; still, check in with your gut instinct and only apply those solutions that you feel good about. When we were ready to sign the papers for the medical laser machine, I had such a strong feeling in the pit of my stomach and a strong whisper, or you may call it an internal voice, told me NOT to sign the papers. I told myself, "Maybe it's your fear holding you back," so I looked at the projections and the research again to satisfy my fear and the numbers looked great. I still had that feeling, though, even as I signed the papers. Does this mean I failed? No, I call it a learning experience because it made me study the industry more thoroughly and I now make decisions by also paying attention to my intuition instead of ignoring it.

Chapter 11

Action

Do not judge me by my successes; judge me by how many times I fell down and got back up again. – Nelson Mandela

There is an old proverb that says human beings are motivated to change when the future looks worse than the present. This proverb reminds me of changes that have taken place very recently in politics. The first is in India where a family dynasty (the Gandhi family) and the Congress Party ruled India for a number of years, but the people of India, especially the poor and today's youth, wanted better jobs, better employment, better education, and less corruption. According to newspapers, the country's vote on May 26, 2014, changed the whole political scene in India by voting in a completely new party and a new prime minister. *The Guardian* quotes, "This is a revolt against India's democratic capitalism, which failed to create sustainable growth beyond 5 percent." The people of India wanted change and could not see that with the Congress Party in power.

The second change in politics is in my own home province of Alberta, Canada, where on May 5, 2015, the people voted for a completely new government after 44 years of Progressive Conservative (PC) Party ruling. The people of Alberta were shocked as well because they expected some change; however, when the PCs came in third, not even in second, that sent a strong message that when Albertans see their future look worse, they are motivated to change.

As human beings, we are motivated to take action because we are in pain or because there is a reward to be had. In both of these examples, people were in pain, and by voting differently, they could already see hope and a reward— improvement in the country or province.

However, there are some of us who are scared of change and will stay where we are for three reasons:

1. It seems unfamiliar to you so you stay inside your comfort zone; or
2. You don't know HOW to move forward ; or
3. You think it's hopeless (believe that you're not capable).

Here's a secret: As you tackle the first two reasons, the third automatically changes from, "It's hopeless and I'm not capable," to "I'm capable and it's worth it!"

In the 2006 movie *The Secret* (featured on *Oprah*), the teachers spoke about *Law of Attraction*. That was the first time I had heard about this universal law, and I was intrigued, but what I felt was missing from it was the idea of taking action. The movie mostly spoke about visualizing your future and being positive, so you manifest easily. The intent of the movie was great, but I believe the message did not come across clearly. In fact, most of my friends who saw the movie and then practiced what the teachers said, never saw any manifestations and felt even more disappointed.

It's a great idea to visualize your awesome future because it creates positive feelings, but nothing will manifest if you don't take action toward making that future become real. Taking action **consistently** is the key to building the future you want.

How do you start taking action? First, by knowing what you want and why you want it. When you go shopping in the mall and are looking for a particular store, you go to the mall directory so you can find your way. The first thing you look for on the mall map is the sign that says, "You are here." Next, you look for the store name and trace it on the map and then you find the easiest way to get there from where you are. Whether you know it or not, you just took a few solid action steps to get from your current state to your desired state.

When I decided I wanted to write a book, I was scared and excited. I was at the You Are Here sign and had no idea where or how to get started, let alone have a finished book in my hand. I was terrified about pouring my life out to strangers and for them to get to know me intimately; plus, I was worried about negative book reviews. This is similar to reason number one, isn't it? The fear of unfamiliarity stops me from stepping out of my comfort zone and keeps me where I am, but something rattled my cage.

One hot summer day, when I was driving from an inspection I had to do on my job as a health inspector, I was lost in thought about my future, and at that time, I knew I wanted to chase after my passion of speaking and sharing my message. The windows were rolled up and the air-conditioning was turned up slightly, but it was serenely quiet as I drove down the lonely highway. I recall talking to myself, in my thoughts, "Zaheen, you have to write a book so it adds to your credibility, but what can you write and speak on specifically?" All of a sudden, and I know this sounds eerie, out of nowhere I heard a whisper in my right ear, *"Fear."* My heart raced as I pulled myself up in my car seat and literally looked in my rear view mirror. As I drove, I tried to dismiss it as my imagination, but I couldn't stop thinking about it. To this day I feel, that just for a second, there was a presence in my car that wanted me to hear that message. I don't know what or who, but that soul-searching rattled my cage, and I knew I had my WHY: all my life I had spent in fear, feeling I didn't have a voice. And up to a few years ago, I still felt I didn't have a voice, and that I wasn't capable. But I kept stretching my comfort zone; I kept visualizing my future as an author and a speaker, and I kept taking action to move toward that goal with small action steps. I want you to find your voice and rise above. I want you to live your life loving fear instead of hating it. I want you to know the endless possibilities outside of your comfort zone, and I want you to know that there is always a way when you are tenacious and ready to improvise.

When you are at a big mall and moving toward your goal of getting to your store, which is on the other side quite a distance away, you may get distracted and go into other stores along the way, but you will get back on route and keep moving toward what you came to do in the first place. You may even stop for a bite to eat at the food court while you collect your thoughts and feed your hunger, but you will then continue on and head toward your store. Similarly, life may present you with a barrier, but you can find a breakthrough and get back on track and move toward a goal if you are passionate about your WHY.

My goal was to have this book completed and to be able to share my message. It took one chapter at a time, but I took action by making the time to write.

Many people ask me, "Zaheen, how are you motivated to write and how did you get motivated to start a wellness centre without a base of clients?" I had a goal, and I have my WHY, but what motivates me is seeing the end result in my head.

With any set goal, a person will be motivated by how the end result makes him or her feel. When I don't feel like exercising, I don't think about the process; I think about how I'll feel after I exercise—energized, clear, and stronger—and this propels me to start exercising. When I go to a restaurant and I'm tempted to eat a bowl of pasta or a burger and fries, I don't think about the process of eating it; I think about how it will make me feel after I've eaten— bloated, sluggish, and gassy—and this stops me from ordering by instant gratification. When I'm selling a service or product to a client, I don't think about the process of selling; I think about meeting the needs of the client.

If you haven't noticed yet, there is a process or system in taking action, and it's very methodical, but it has to be practiced so it becomes unconscious. There are three steps to taking action:

1. Know your WHY
2. Visualize your end result
3. Think about the consequences of taking or NOT taking actions

For example, when I was struggling with my weight, I decided it was time to change my relationship with food. My WHY involved having peace of mind, feeling confident, and having energy instead of the constant mind battle about food or feeling worthless. I visualized the end result of me being at my ideal weight and being happy with myself. But I also had to think about the consequences of taking action or NOT taking action because it made me aware of my patterns and behaviors in that context. Here are some questions that can help you figure out the cost of your consequences:

Consequence Questions (adapted from NLP):

1. What is the best thing that can happen if I take this step?
2. What is the worst thing that can happen if I take this step?

3. What is the best thing that can happen if I don't take this step?

4. What's the worst thing that can happen if I don't take this step?

Once you use these steps of knowing your WHY, visualizing the end result and considering your consequences, then you have lit the fire in your belly to take action!

You'll hear resilient people say, "Success is about taking consistent actions." You may not see the pay off immediately, but these little action steps add up. My mentor, Michael Losier, says, "Stay in line and keep doing what you are doing because your turn will come, and you will be standing in front of that line someday." Just as resilience and success are two sides of a coin, so are passion and sacrifice. If you are passionate about what you want, and you want to be a difference-maker, there are times that you will have to sacrifice what's dearest to you for a short time.

When I wrote this book, I'd wake up every Sunday morning and write between 5 and 11 am because that is the only time I had available to write. I sacrificed sleep, and I sacrificed time with my family on Sunday mornings for a few months as I completed my book, but I took consistent action every week to reach my goal.

One piece of advice as you take action toward your goal is to learn how to improvise. Resilience is not about achieving your goal; it's about the journey to a destination because you start mastering yourself by becoming aware of strengths and weaknesses. Improvisation is about being flexible and being able to adapt to circumstances as you strive toward what you want. As an entrepreneur, I'm constantly improvising my marketing and my message. After every keynote speech or workshop, I have a "light bulb" moment of something I used earlier that could work brilliantly in the next keynote or workshop. After every marketing campaign and learning from the data analytics, I learn what worked and what did not work, and I ask myself how I can make it better next time.

Therefore, to be action-oriented you have to remember three things:

- Think/behave like a slinky—be flexible, adaptable, stretch outside your comfort zone, and know you can bounce back.

- Think/behave like your GPS (or Google Maps)—even if you get a curve ball or get stuck in your journey toward your goal, find another way to get to your destination by improvising.

- Think/behave like a rolling snowball—become aware of what you are good at and build on your strengths in that area.

Chapter 12

Passion & Purpose

*Every mighty king was once a crying baby! Every great tree was once a
tiny seed! Every tall building was once in paper! And so I dream my
dream.*

– Eunice Akoth

Emmanuel Jal, a former child soldier from South Sudan, is
now a recording artist and a peace activist. After being sent
to the front lines and forced to do many unimaginable,
horrible things between the ages of 8 and 13, Jal and a group
of young boys escaped the camp in Ethiopia and walked for
thousands of miles to return home. Tired and hungry, many
died. Jal became so desperate that at one point he nearly
succumbed to cannibalism. Jal ended up in a town called
Waat, where he met Emma McCune. The British aid worker
was working for Street Kids International, a UNICEF-
funded Canadian charity that built and renovated schools in
southern Sudan; she smuggled Jal onto an aid flight to
Kenya. She put him into school and eventually adopted him.
Sadly, six months after arriving in Nairobi, McCune was
killed in a car accident. Jal now uses his music to spread the

word of peace, and in fact, in his bio, he states, "I believe I survived for a reason…to tell my story and touch lives." This is the story of a thriver—a person who thrives—because he decided to have a purpose in life. Jal's purpose is very clear to him: *Shine a light where there's darkness.*

Malala Yousafzai is a Pakistani activist for female education and the youngest ever Nobel Prize laureate. She rose against the Taliban in her native town in Pakistan because they banned girls from attending school. One afternoon in October 2012, as she was boarding the school bus, a gunman fired three shots, one of which hit her forehead. She was only 15 years old at the time, and she still fights for girls' rights to education. This is another story of a thriver.

Tricia Downing, an avid cyclist, drove across the country in the summer of 2000 for what amounted to eighteen races in twenty-three days. She returned from her adventure to a fresh start. A new job awaited her, but on September 17, 2000, Tricia Downing's life took a detour. While training on her bicycle one sunny Colorado afternoon, Tricia collided with a car that turned directly in her path, and she was instantly paralyzed from the chest down. As a competitive road and track cyclist and lifelong athlete, losing the use of her legs was devastating on all accounts. As she re-learns to do everything from sitting up straight to navigating through her house in a wheelchair to returning to work and operating a hand cycle, her grueling recovery takes her to the very core of her athletic mettle. This inner strength helps her to not only learn how to live life as a paraplegic—a label that takes time to grow accustomed to—but to have the courage to return to the competitive sport she loves and almost lost. Determined to live life on her terms, Tricia turned her misfortune into opportunity, becoming a world-class wheelchair racer, author, and speaker, and she founded her own camp for other women in similar situations. Tricia is a thriver.

I can share many stories of resilient individuals who just keep thriving, and these are not peace activists or famous celebrities but individuals like you and me who live their passion and purpose instead of just getting by. That is the difference! There are individuals who have survived traumas, financial losses, addictions, and war, but they keep living, turning their fear and struggle into a purpose. When survivors turn that pain into a purpose, it's called THRIVING. Even though memories may haunt them or a hint of weakness could lead them off their path, this burning desire to their purpose keeps them thriving.

There are also individuals who believe in your purpose even when you can't see it—they become the fire in your belly, and they help you see your purpose. I call these people *resilient angels* because they are by your side while you thrive, and they sense and see your purpose in the world.

I recently watched a movie depicting the life story of Sir Ludwig Guttman, a Jewish doctor who fled Nazi Germany just before the start of the Second World War. Guttman reminds me of a *resilient angel* because he is considered to be one of the founding fathers of Paralympics. During the war when soldiers came into his infirmary missing a body part or having a spinal injury, most had given up on living. However, Guttman believed that sport was a major method of therapy for injured military personnel, helping them build up physical strength and self-respect. He noticed that the soldiers started to not only get stronger, but they started to regain hope of living a life of possibility. Guttman organized the first paraplegic games in 1948, which later went on to become known as the Paralympics.

In 2006, while on maternity leave from my job as a public health inspector, a friend came to my house and introduced me to a great skin care line. I had never heard about multi-level marketing or network marketing, and she explained how I could make money selling skin care and building a business by recruiting others to sell. I tried the products for a week and instantly fell in love with them, but I was apprehensive about doing small presentations in people's houses. First, I felt I was incapable of selling anything, and second, I was so scared of stuttering while I presented that I wondered who would purchase from me, let alone join me in this endeavor.

As I read through the company information, I remember telling myself, "Zaheen, public speaking is one of the fears you want to accomplish, and it's on your bucket list. This may be a good way to start." I jumped in with both feet and practiced the presentation. As I started to offer brief presentations in other people's homes and in front of strangers, I realized I enjoyed public speaking! I'd receive compliments from customers who bought from me because I showed enthusiasm, I was transparent with my message, I believed in what I was selling, and I only gave them what they wanted at that time to meet their needs.

The following year, the skin care network marketing company was having a conference in Atlanta, and a few of us decided to go. I remember sitting in a stadium-like arena and my friend Gaye, who introduced me to these products, sat next to me. The first keynote presenter walked up to the huge stage with a walking cane—he was blind. During his keynote speech, he talked about his passion for mountain climbing and showed us pictures of him climbing Mount

Everest! I kept thinking to myself, "Here's a guy who's not letting his disability stop him from climbing mountains, and here I am worried about a simple thing like a stutter!" I felt sorry for him, yet I was in awe because even though he loved climbing, he couldn't see breathtaking views from the mountain top or even see his own pictures, yet he did not complain. His message was simple: *Don't let anything stop you from doing what you want.*

I turned to Gaye and said, "You know, I could be on that stage. I've realized I like sharing my knowledge and inspiring others."

"Zaheen, I know you can, and you'd be so great at it," Gaye replied, giving me a boost of confidence.

On the same day, during lunch, Gaye and I went to a small bookstore, and I asked the store clerk if they had any books by Les Brown or Brian Tracy other than the couple on the shelves. The store clerk went into the back to look and then emerged with a book in her hand to say, "Ma'am this is the only book I had in the back." As she handed me the book, and I read the title, time slowed down almost to a standstill, and the chatter in the background became muffled. My heart stopped for a second, and I stopped breathing as I read the title: *Speak to Win* by Brian Tracy. I took a deep breath and felt flushed. Is this a sign? Even though this wasn't the book

I was looking for, it was the only book the store clerk handed me. At that moment, I knew I had to pursue this calling no matter what—I had found my purpose.

I turned my pain of stuttering into a purpose, especially when I saw my little angel daughter, Arissa, sleeping in her crib on my return from Atlanta. As she slept peacefully and I looked lovingly at her, it hit me that she will look up at me as her role model. Her mom had usually avoided speaking situations, her mom lived in fear, and even after knowing her purpose, she ignored it. What kind of role model would I be to my daughter?

Do I want to teach her to ignore her gifts? Do I want to teach her to live in fear and silence? Do I want her to be in a career that is not satisfying just because everyone else thinks she SHOULD be a lawyer or doctor or engineer? No.

I want my daughter to have a voice, and I want her to stretch her comfort zone so she can continue to learn more about herself. I want her to shine in her light and bathe in that light because then she will feel the most fulfilled.

As I saw her sleeping peacefully, my conviction grew because she became the fire in my belly. Similarly, the children in South Sudan became the fire in Emmanuel Jal's belly, the girls of Pakistan became the fire in Malala

Yousafzai's belly, and disabled athletic women became the fire in Tricia Downing's belly.

From then on, I chose to live my life thriving instead of complaining and playing the victim. A thriver is someone who transforms his or her pain (emotional or physical) into something positive and adapts to whatever life sends because in their minds, they know that as a result of this struggle, something positive will occur. Some people call this mental toughness, I call it "thriving to build resilience." Thriving is not about being strong; it's about everyday coping skills and your reaction to the event (read chapter on emotional resilience for coping skills). Thriving is about living with your passion and your purpose; a person needs both.

You may be asking, "I don't know what my purpose or passion is, and I haven't gone through traumatic events like Emmanuel, Malala, or Tricia, so how do I find that passion and purpose?" My mentor, Lisa Nichols, one of the teachers in the movie *Secret*, whom I have heard speak numerous times and have taken her World Class Speaking Alliance (WCSA) year-long program, explains it very well. She says, "Life happens in stages and at each stage, we are called to move into our next life assignment; we do that by listening to our intuitive self or to that pull in your belly that draws you toward your passion."

121

I didn't know that I had a voice, let alone that I'd become a speaker! But life happens in stages. First, I was introduced to ISTAR (Institute of Stuttering Treatment and Research) and I started to make changes in my belief systems by practicing the skills that I acquired. Second, I became a public health inspector where I felt I was making a difference in public health. Third, I was introduced to network marketing (I don't practice anymore), which empowered me with a new belief and propelled me into the speaking industry. Lastly, I became an owner of a wellness centre with my husband, Badur, which allows us to create transformation and healing in other people's lives.

Where has life taken you? Is it beckoning you toward working with teenagers, seniors, or even bettering the environment? Is your belly pulling you toward starting a business? Is your intuition pushing you toward a leadership or management position because it's time? Stop ignoring your inner voice and ask yourself, "Where can I start or who can I ask for help in guiding me toward my passion and purpose?"

If you're still unsure of your passion or purpose, let's break it down so you understand it better:

Passion: What do you like to do? What do enjoy doing so much that you are not watching the clock? I'm not talking about hobbies and playing video games. I'm talking about where you feel fulfilled, where you find you are making a difference. What kinds of things did you like doing as a child or teenager before you were told what you SHOULD do? Did you like art, did you like a particular sport, or did you like writing or being creative in a different way? My passion is to share my message about being resilient in life and business. My husband's passion is massage therapy, and he'd massage his friends without charging a fee to relieve their pain.

Purpose: Why do you want to do it? What do you get out of pursuing your passion? My purpose is two-fold: The first is to be a role-model to my daughter, and the second is the knowledge that if I can help one person or business bounce back, then I've made a difference. My husband's purpose is to heal and better the health of his clients, and if he can do so, then he has made a difference.

If you love your career, then that is your passion, and if you have a calling to help others, then find a way to volunteer in an organization that's in alignment with your cause. Only then are you thriving and finding an outlet to channel your purpose and feeling fulfilled at the same time. You can't have passion without purpose, and you can't have purpose without passion.

Emmanuel Jal uses his music (his passion) as a platform to provide children an opportunity to get an education (his purpose). Malala Yousafzai uses her story and her foundation, the Malala Fund (passion), as a platform to educate girls in Pakistan (purpose). Tricia Downing uses her athletic platform as a wheelchair racer (passion) to help other disabled women (purpose).

A great resource for discovering your passion and life purpose is *The Passion Test* by Janet and Chris Attwood. Visit their website and take their FREE assessment: http://www.thepassiontest.com/take-the-passion-test/personal-passion-profile-2/

Chapter 13

Attitude

I'm not what has happened to me. I'm what I choose to become.

– Carl Jung

My mentors, Tim and Kris Hallbom, travel the world teaching neuro linguistic programming (NLP), and in 2001, they were invited to Sydney, Australia, to teach their program. They decided to go early and stay an extra week so they could spend some time in Cairns and finish in Port Douglas, a beautiful island. The day arrived when they had to leave Port Douglas for Sydney. During the cab ride to the local airport, Kris said to the cab driver, "This island is so beautiful. How I envy those who live here!"

The driver replied, "You're Americans, I can tell from the accent. Yes, it's beautiful, but it's only for rich folks." However, he went on to tell them how lucky they were because the economy in Australia wasn't that great, and he didn't make enough money even though he drove the cab six days a week. The only time he had fun was on Sundays when he got together with his buddies to drink and flip burgers in his backyard. And this went on until they arrived at the local airport to catch their flight into Sydney.

After arriving in Sydney, they stepped outside the airport to get a cab to drive them to the hotel. Within seconds, a cab pulled up and the driver hopped out, cheerfully greeting them and helping them with the luggage.

"Where you from?" the driver asked.

"California, USA," Tim replied.

"Is this your first time to Sydney?" he asked.

"Yes, but it's not a holiday," one of them replied.

"How about if I take you on a longer ride to your hotel so you can see some sites, and I will not charge you extra," the driver suggested. Tim and Kris were delighted and agreed right away.

During the ride, Kris started telling the driver they had spent some time in Cairns, finishing off in Port Douglas and how they really enjoyed the beautiful island. The driver replied, "Oh that is where the wife and I are going to retire in a couple of months." Tim and Kris looked at each other in surprise because this island is known for its million-dollar houses. Being curious, they asked the driver how he was going to do that.

He said, "My house in Sydney is worth a lot more now, and we don't owe anything on it. I've made some investments thanks to some advice I got from clients in my back seat, and so the wife and I have enough money to retire," he explained.

"Are you going to miss what you do?" Tim asked.

"I'll miss driving my cab. I've been driving a cab for 30 years," he replied.

This story features two men with the same job in the same economy, but consider how differently they saw life and their futures. The first driver hated what he did and probably did nothing about it, while the second driver loved his work and thought about his future!

Which one would you want to hang out with?

Have you walked into a store or business looking for some service, but received poor service and a negative attitude instead? How did that experience make you feel?

In your own work or business, how is your attitude toward your staff, your customers, or clients? Do you take that extra care to make them feel important? The second cab driver did that by offering a longer ride to Tim and Kris—no wonder he got great advice from people in his back seat on how to invest his money!

Mistakes are going to be made, setbacks are going to occur, and losses are bitter, but don't let that affect your attitude because it will drag you down. If you face life knowing that you have the coping skills and that there's something positive in every mistake, every setback, and every loss, then whatever comes your way will be easier to handle because you are already thinking of ways to handle it—and you will look for that learning lesson so you can incorporate it the next time.

I realized that only I could help myself if I wanted to speak effortlessly and be able to express my ideas. Instead of having a negative attitude of "nothing works" or "speech therapy was a waste of time," I decided to have a positive attitude and use the skills I received to give it a try. I knew I wouldn't be fluent the first time, I'd make mistakes, and experience setbacks, but I kept on trying, using baby steps and taking something positive away from each experience. When the equipment we bought for our centre wasn't making us money like we thought it would, I developed a negative attitude toward the industry and the town we lived in, but I quickly realized that it was up to me to turn this around and make it profitable.

I've spent thousands of dollars on courses, training, and coaching. Sometimes one pays thousands of dollars for coaching or a training course only to realize not much new was gained. This has happened to me, too! However, I don't regret spending all that money because there's always a good takeaway no matter what.

When I decided to publish my first book, *Attract Your Ideal Weight: 8 Secrets of People Who Lose Weight and Keep It Off,* I decided to go with a publisher that was offering a great deal but I never looked into their history. I was told my books would be ready by February, but after numerous phone calls and threatening to pull my contract, I finally got my books in June. Later, I found out that the publishing company had done similar things to other authors.

They say things happen for a reason. During May and June, our community was raising money for a little girl who had a brain tumor, and this surgery could only be done by a neurosurgeon in Texas. The family's projected costs ran to $250,000. My husband and I wanted to support the family somehow through our company, Shanti Wellness Centre, Inc. I decided to have a book launch party in a restaurant and asked the restaurant to sponsor the meal and space, while all proceeds from book sales and a silent auction would go toward raising funds for this little girl. Now when I look back, I'm glad my books were delayed until June. This insight helped me remember that no matter what happens—

mistakes, setbacks, or losses—there's always something positive in it.

In my research of resilient and successful people, I've found that a positive attitude is a common theme, but what *is* a positive attitude? It encompasses these five traits:

1. Optimism. All the research on optimism says that people who are optimistic are happier, have great relationships, are healthier, and are good at problem solving. However, what makes a person happier? I've seen resilient entrepreneurs happier because they maximize their strengths and accomplishments and know that if they use their strengths in challenging business decisions, it could lead to a better situation; that is optimism. I've seen couples or business partners flourish in relationships because they maximize what makes them best at what they do thereby complementing each other. Karen Reivich, Ph.D., author of *The Resilience Factor: 7 Keys to Finding Your Inner Strength and Overcoming Life's Hurdles,* explains it best, "Resilient people rely on their strengths to navigate the challenges in life."

2. Sense of Humor. Laughter is the best medicine and it has been proven by Dr. Madhan Kataria, founder of Laughter Yoga and SVYASA in Bangalore, India, one of the world's leading yoga research organizations. Two hundred participants were randomly selected from three Bangalore IT companies and divided into two groups: control group and laughter yoga group. After seven laughter yoga sessions over 18 days, researchers found a 6 percent reduction in systolic blood pressure and a 4 percent reduction in diastolic blood pressure, indicating reduced stress levels and relaxation. Cortisol is a stress hormone that accurately reflects perceived stress levels. In this study, the laughter yoga group had a 28 percent reduction in cortisol compared to 16 percent in the control group. Finally, The PANAS (Positive Affectivity and Negative Affectivity Scale) test assesses the "emotional style" a person uses to cope with events in their life. There was a 27 percent decrease in negative emotions in the laughter yoga group and no significant change in the control group. This research demonstrates that being able to laugh at life's frustrations could increase immunity, and in turn, create a positive attitude. Look for a laughter yoga club in your area.

3. Flexibility. In neuro linguistic programing (NLP), there are some key pre-suppositions:

a) *If what you are doing is not working, do something different.* It sounds so simple, yet you don't always feel it's necessary to change your behaviour. I have clients who wish they could change their spouse or business partner and my answer to them is, "I can't help you with that, but I can help you with changing yourself first." This pre-supposition is about changing strategies instead of beating one's head against the wall, but first a person needs to become aware of what's not working.

b) *The person with the most flexibility will have more control.* When one views a challenge and comes up with several different ways to handle it, that demonstrates flexibility in trying different methods to overcome this challenge, and this keeps a person more in control of a situation. This way of thinking also leads to a positive attitude.

4. Embrace Change. Joseph O'Connor, author of *Free Yourself from Fears with NLP*, explains that change occurs through external forces (outside our control) or internally (you decide to make the change). When change occurs externally, your first reaction is anxiety because you've lost something of value and are not sure if you can replace it. In addition, with change comes uncertainty; however, when one makes the change internally, he or she feels more in control because the resources will be on hand, or they will seek out the resources necessary to make the change easier. O'Connor further states that any change is the balancing act between two forces: the magnitude of the challenge and the resources we feel we have to deal with it. Therefore, embracing change becomes easier when you have or seek out the resources you need and when you understand the value behind change because it may help you to let go of the old while bringing in the new.

5. Realistic. Being optimistic must also involve being realistic, because it doesn't help when you ignore the problems that exist. Holocaust survivors and prisoners of war had realistic optimism because even though they were distressed and acknowledged that

133

they may never be rescued (realistic), they took each day of survival and each bit of good news with optimism. In life and business, a person will face some harsh realities, but when you maximize your strengths in that area, you will find optimism.

Having and cultivating a positive attitude is key in building resilience. I'm not saying you don't have a positive attitude now; I'm saying that just like me, you too can be faced with challenges or life situations where you can ignore that you're responding negatively to others and to yourself. Having the system to quickly bounce back involves remembering the 5 traits of building a positive attitude.

Cultivating resilient traits in life and business is more important now than ever before with changing economies, new technologies, and a new generation emerging. Every day we hear about a new app or a new way to market our services, and we have to keep up with this trend. It's not going to go away. There are times that you may feel overwhelmed or frustrated; I know I do. However, these four principles, which are found in resilient individuals and organizations, will help you get through in life and business. I also call it POOP (it's not what you think!):

Plan ahead. When we decided to open up the wellness centre, we had to face a few harsh realities, the first being that we would not get a truckload of customers walking in on day one. This is a service industry, and it takes time to build customers' trust when it comes to their health and wellness. Second, we may not retain the therapists or practitioners forever because they could move away or decide to work from home. Here's a list of what we did to overcome the first challenge:

1. Advertise in the local paper, have a website, and have a social media presence.

2. Build an email list and sending out regular emails to our clients.

3. Have an Open House a month after we started and offer a preview of our services for a minimal price with an upsell of enticing packages.

4. Offer seasonal and monthly specials through our email subscriber list.

5. Door-to-door campaign with a marketing company a year after we opened without adding any of our own capital.

These actions alone grew our customer base by 200 percent in six months, and referrals started coming in! We were nominated Best Business of The Year in 2014, just four years after we opened our doors.

If faced with a challenging situation in life and business, do the following:

a) Make a list of things that could go wrong.

b) Make a list of your strengths.

c) Make a list of the resources you could tap into to help you with the task at hand.

Obstacle mastery. Now look at the list of things that could go wrong and for each one ask, "What strategies could I implement here?" Don't come up with just one; think of two or three. This is about having flexibility so that you feel more in control. Now look at the list of your strengths, resources, and strategies together, highlighting the strategy that correlates closely with the strengths and resources you currently have. You have just incorporated the first step in taking action and mastering your obstacle.

Outcome orientation. Richard Wiseman conducted a large study showing the importance of the way we approach goals. He tracked 5,000 people who had some significant goal they wanted to achieve. He found that the successful goal setters described their goal in **positive terms** and considered carefully what **challenges they would face** actually doing the work to achieve it. Wiseman further explained that the successful ones were able to list concrete specific benefits they would get from achieving their goal. In one of his examples, he said, "They wrote them down and explained what each benefit could bring, like enjoying two evenings with friends and visiting one new country each year."

Now, make a list of specific benefits for the strategy that you chose in **Obstacle mastery** and notice the outcome you desire.

Pattern recognition. Becoming aware of your subconscious patterns that sabotage your success or keep you stuck is the most important step in cultivating a positive attitude, embracing change, and bouncing back from challenges. I had a pattern where I'd get upset easily when someone pointed out the truth and I'd walk away thinking that they were wrong and I was right. But that pattern bothered me. Why couldn't I just accept what the person was saying to me? I realized that pattern was a defense mechanism because I wanted to prove that I was smart, that I knew it all and that my opinion mattered. Once I realized the positive intent of my behavior and recognized this pattern, I consciously started making changes by listening and understanding their perspective.

Do you have a pattern that sabotages your success or keeps you stuck? Ask the following questions:

a) What is the purpose of this pattern?

b) If I continue this pattern what will happen?

c) What can I do differently next time I recognise this pattern?

d) What will be the evidence that I have broken this pattern?

Chapter 14

Relationships Skills

When you really listen to another person from their point of view, and reflect back to them that understanding, it's like giving them emotional oxygen.

— Stephen Covey

Resilient individuals create a supportive network and are apt at handling and reducing conflict because they've learned the intricate language and skills of building and maintaining relationships. Communication skills and relationship building is not only about listening and respect—it's significantly more than that. It involves a subconscious contract of understanding the other person's perspective and intention. Think of a leader or manager whom you admire and notice how he or she interacts with you or with others at all levels in the company or when networking. You will notice the following, and the easiest way to remember this is LIMP:

- **L**isten: She's listening for words that indicate the person's communication style and then communicates back using that style.

- **I**ntention: She is listening for the person's underlying reason.

- **M**atch and mirror: She subconsciously picks up the opposite person's body language, tone of voice, and information style (detail or big picture), and mirrors that.

- **P**erspective: She behaves respectfully and shows genuine interest in what's important to the other person.

When you follow the theory of LIMP and practice the skills, you will create great rapport, be a master at reducing conflict, positively influence others, and have a supportive network around you.

Rapport involves creating a harmonious relationship that works in both directions, where you may have differing opinions, but those opinions are respected and working relationships are improved.

Conflict occurs because you are not following any or all of the aspects of LIMP. As a public health inspector, I was faced with conflict almost every day, but as my supervisor said, I have a knack for handling challenging situations and calming others down. One day, I went into a restaurant, a well-known franchise, to conduct an inspection. After I was finished, I asked for the owner, whom I was meeting for the first time, and from the moment he saw me, his demeanor became agitated and he avoided eye contact. As I explained my findings in a calm voice, he became more upset, so I stopped what I was saying. I said, "Sir, let's rewind. I'm going to go out the door, walk in again and ask for you first, then introduce myself and we'll have a chat about how you're doing and only then will I go through my findings. How does that sound?" I said.

He looked at me, smiled and said, "You don't need to do that; I'll take care of what you've pointed out." Clearly, when he saw me, he only saw "Public Health Inspector with Enforcement Stick and Bad News"; he didn't see Zaheen Nanji. On the other hand, I never made it a point to create rapport with him before going through my findings; instead, I was breaking rapport. Over the years, I have come to realize that I get more compliance from operators when I build rapport with them and follow LIMP.

The same is true as a business owner. Our client loyalty comes from practicing and implementing LIMP. Recently, I was involved in a car accident and was looking at purchasing another vehicle. I went to four different dealerships where I noticed that every salesperson had a different approach. Two of the four showed me the newest models and promotions of the month, while never asking me about my buying criteria. The only criteria they asked for was my budget. One of the four completely broke rapport with me by making me sit down and fill out a form with my name and contact information and then asked about my budget while looking at his computer screen; finally, he took us out to show us one model. The last salesperson had superb LIMP skills even though I did not end up purchasing a car. He asked a few questions, listened, asked about my buying criteria, and then matched a couple of models. Then he took me onto the lot to show me similar models because he did not have the exact one on site. Even though I did not get to test drive a car, I felt comfortable with him because he created great rapport with me, and he made it a point to connect with me at another level by asking more about how that car would fit into my lifestyle.

Here I further break down LIMP into tools that you can implement right away:

1. Listen. Human beings receive and communicate information in four main communication styles, but one style is the preferred or dominant style:

a) Visual: You learn by watching or having images. You think in pictures and like to see your way clearly so you have a long-term vision, but you tend to skip details and are impatient. You use words such as clear, focus, look, see, clarity, show, picture, visualize.

b) Auditory: You learn by listening or talking it out. You brainstorm ideas and are detailed when explaining a project, but you get upset when interrupted. You use words such as sound, hear, tune, resonate, idea, listen, repeat.

c) Kinesthetic: You learn by doing and feeling. You connect well with others and make decisions based on how you feel. You like keeping a balance, but you dislike too many choices. You use words such as comfortable, feel, fits, grasp, connect, get, touch.

d) Digital: You learn by having facts and figures. You solve problems and prioritize well, but you can also be stubborn. You use words such as think, makes sense, figure it, process it, first, second, list.

Whether you are conversing, networking, selling, or coaching, listen to the words and phrases the other person is using and converse back in their preferred style.

2. Intention. What is the other's person intention or their underlying aim, rather than what they are saying? The positive intention behind the restaurant owner's agitated behaviour was that he was worried I

was going to either shut down his restaurant, or I'd hurt his ego by telling him how unsanitary his operation was. Either way, I had to understand the underlying aim behind his behaviour instead of confronting him and making the situation worse. Similarly, when you are in conflict with a client or co-worker, ask yourself, "What is he/she trying to gain out of this behaviour?" Most often when a discussion turns into an argument, the underlying aim of the person yelling is that she feels unheard, or she feels she's lost control and wants to gain it back.

3. Match and mirror. There has been ample research on how body language can reveal much about what a person is communicating. How one gestures, his or her body posture, and facial expressions can either build or break rapport. Recall the last time you had a live conversation with your best friend. I'm sure you didn't even notice how you leaned in to talk or made the same facial expressions and laughed. You were becoming in sync with each other and understanding each other's world. When creating rapport, match body postures and gestures, breathing rates and voice tonality and speed. However, when reducing conflict, pace by first listening and acknowledging the other person and then lead by making your voice calmer,

144

speaking at a slower speed, and slowing down breathing.

4. Perspective. To really understand the other person's perspective, you have to figuratively step into their shoes. Hostage negotiators are trained to step into the hostage-taker's shoes to not only understand his underlying aim but to understand the whole situation and predict the next move. In short, it's about understanding the other person rather than the other person understanding YOU. When someone is telling us a problem, often we voice our own problem at the same time and forget about the other person's. Instead, listen and step into her shoes and really understand her situation. Recall the last time you had an argument with a significant other or business partner. Now, be there and float out of your own body and observe the situation as a third person. Then, float into the other person and look at you from his eyes and feel what he's feeling. Finally, float out and back into your body. Now that you have the perspective as a third person and as the other involved person, how would you handle this situation the next time around?

As I write this book, I've been happily married for 15 years, and my husband and I have been business partners for 5 years. When we get together for family reunions, we get teased about how happy we are in each other's company, and we truly enjoy being in each other's company. Our clients often comment on our great working relationship as business partners, and they're always asking us for tips on how to make it work. We've consciously used LIMP with each other, and now it's become so subconscious that we understand each other's intention and perspective and automatically communicate in each other's style as well. More than that, we respect each other's areas of strength and allow each to explore and gain more knowledge in that area.

As a speaker, facilitator, and leader, you need to connect with your audience by using the keywords and principles from all four styles of communication. Have images for the visual person on your handouts or presentations; have some emotion and stories for the kinesthetic person; and, have the audience partner up or do group work for the auditory person, and have some facts and figures for the digital person.

Resilient people also know how to break rapport discreetly without completely offending the other person. The easiest way to do that is to stop matching and mirroring and by knowing your boundaries. Then, you can change voice tone and speed, stop gesturing, break eye contact, or even use facial expressions. For example, here's what I do to break rapport without severing relationships:

1. Workload. If I have deadlines to meet or a heavy workload, I'll make it clear I have some demands to meet and will give the person a time or day that we can meet or chat some more. Don't be afraid to use boundaries because people will respect you and your time more as long as long you don't ignore them.

2. Closing a sale. There is a process to making a sale, and when I have given the client the information they need, I'll give them some space so they can process it and invite them again to ask any more questions. If I'm on the phone, I'll tell them to weigh the information and I'll give them a few minutes before closing the deal. Here I'm breaking rapport slightly to avoid the buyer feeling guilty and severing a long-term client relationship, because once remorse sets in, they may not come back again.

3. Breaking away by asking permission. When I'm at a networking event and speaking with a person who has been talking about her business or life and doesn't know when to stop, I'll say, "Would you

mind if I go talk to that lady over there because she has something I'd like to ask her about?" You'll never hear them say no.

As resilient people create rapport, they also create a supportive network or client loyalty. Whenever resilient people need some help in getting a project done or are looking for volunteers, it is their supportive network that comes to their aid.

Chapter 15

Appreciation

I'm thankful for my struggle because without it, I wouldn't have stumbled across my strength.

– Alex Elle

When resilient individuals are faced with challenges, they have two streams of thought running through their minds: one is about finding solutions and the other is about all the things they appreciate in life. It's as though there is a subconscious REFRAME button they push whenever their thoughts and emotions turn to worry and fear, because after a short time, they've perked up and are more positive and appreciative about what they already have. They were not born with this ability, but they were taught by other influencers; they have trained themselves to look at what they already have rather than stewing in worry.

Resilient individuals get worried and overwhelmed just like everyone else, but it's this one subconscious step of appreciation they implement that completely makes them flip the coin on the challenges they face and makes them feel more hopeful.

All the research on holocaust survivors and prisoners of war show that the conscious practice of appreciating each day of survival and each morsel of food, instead of thinking about dying, got them through the day. Louis "Louie" Zamperini was an American prisoner of war survivor in World War II and an Olympic distance runner. His life story has been featured in a biography and in the movie *Unbroken*. What struck me about his story is not the fact that he survived being in a Japanese POW camp, which was brutal, but the 47 days he spent stranded at sea with two army officers. They were subjected to the unrelenting sun, runs by Japanese bombers, circling sharks, and little drinking water. To survive, they collected rainwater and killed birds that happened to land on the raft or they caught fish and ate it raw. One of the men died at sea before Zamperini and the plane's pilot, Russell Allen "Phil" Phillips, finally washed ashore. They found themselves on a Pacific island 2000 miles from the crash site and in enemy Japanese territory.

Spending a month and half at sea under these conditions would have broken a lot of men, but somehow Zamperini and Phillips only thought about how to survive each day and to appreciate the little things, such as each other's company, the inedible raw food, and the fact they were still alive. What kept them going was not the negative loop of, "What if I don't make it," but the positive story that read, "We will be rescued soon."

Once a thriving successful business woman, my mother lost most of it in 2010. She was 66 years old. At that age, most are thinking about retirement and enjoying rewards that were planted throughout life. My parents had worked hard in the bakery business and had implemented systems where things ran smoothly, and they could semi-retire. The business was left in capable hands of managers.

After learning that the business was losing money and that she owed millions of shillings (Kenyan currency) in bank loans and to various suppliers, she was devastated. In the process of fixing this, she sold all her assets except for one piece of land on which she has her bakery now, and she promised to pay the remaining monies in installments that she owed to her suppliers. As I write this book, she is almost 70 years old and still runs her own bakery, and still she owes some money. She has paid back most of her debt.

Recently, I spoke to her on the phone about this and asked, "Mom, you are 70 years old, and you say you're enjoying life, yet you work and you still owe money. How can you be so positive?"

"I was devastated and cried for weeks, but then I was able to pull through. Yes, I still owe lots of money, but the debt is going to go away, someday. I don't worry about that; instead, I look at what I already have. I'm 70 years old, but I feel like I'm only 60. At this age, most women I know sit at home and may have nothing to look forward to, but I do. I spend half a day at work and I enjoy that; I spend Tuesdays playing cards with my friends and Sunday afternoon going to the movies. I volunteer in our community and lead some committees because I enjoy it. I'm enjoying my life and I'm not depending on anyone for it."

My mother has implanted that subconscious reframe button and she keeps practicing the act of appreciation, which is the ability to look at what you already have rather than being worried about what you don't have.

I was at a conference in California during the month that Baltimore was in chaos. Freddie Gray, a 25-year-old African American resident of Baltimore, Maryland, sustained injuries following his arrest by policemen. Gray died on April 19, 2015, after going into a coma.

At this conference, I was sharing a hotel room with another conference participant that I had only met on Facebook; I'll call her Mary. Mary is an African-American. From the time she arrived, her eyes were glued to the CNN channel, and during that time, CNN kept showing the riots in Baltimore. As she watched the news, she got more depressed and angry and wished she hadn't come to the conference. I asked her why she felt that way, and she told me how she had lost both her young adult sons in one day, and that these riots were bringing back memories. She went on to explain that fateful day to me where one son died of natural health causes in the morning and the other son was shot in the back by a police officer that afternoon. I couldn't imagine what she had to go through to mourn not one but two children dying from different circumstances. She had braced herself for the son she knew would not survive because of his health condition, but nothing had prepared her for the more immediate loss of the second boy.

Mary sought justice for wrongful arrest and the death of her son, and she won. She became a celebrity in her own town, and she was featured on the news. As she showed me the news clip of her being interviewed after she had won the case, I saw a woman who was strong, standing tall, at peace, and who believed in her cause.

"Mary," I said, "when I see that clip, I see someone who has been able to hold herself with integrity even after losing two sons on the same day. You fought for justice, and you got it. The Mary I see here today feels like she has lost again and she's angry. Why? I know it brings back memories, but what's going on?"

She answered, "A part of me thinks, what if I had been there and was able to stop my son from getting shot, but I know if I had not been at the hospital either, I'd not have spent the last moments with my sick son. A part of me gets angry that our African-American sons are targeted, and why can't this stop? We [African-American mothers] are always scared when our sons go out, hoping they aren't wrongfully arrested. I just want this to stop," Mary replied with a sigh of sadness.

"What do you appreciate about your sons and this whole experience you had?" I asked

"I was told that my sick son would not live past his seventh birthday, but he lived into his early twenties and also became a father himself. I'm glad he got to live his life into adulthood. I'm glad that the justice system was on my side, and my other son's reputation remained intact."

"Mary, people need to hear your story, and instead of getting angry and feeling negative when you turn to the news channel, appreciate what you had and what that experience has taught and given you. You are not going to get your sons back, but your experience can help other mothers and their sons. Take your mess and turn into a message for others," I replied softly yet assertively.

Mary's eyes widened and she sat up straight. She told me how she needed to hear this, and she'd work toward her purpose. After that conversation, Mary's demeanor became more positive, more hopeful, and appreciative toward being at the conference.

At any given time during your daily activities, your mind is bombarded with millions of bits of sensory stimulations from the physical environment—sounds, smells, tastes, sights, and feelings are continually being downloaded into your system, and your mind needs a way to filter that information.

The reticular activating system (RAS) sits at the base of your brain and includes the part of the brain stem to the base of the spinal cord; it acts as a filter that adapts to different situations based on your belief system. However, these sensory downloads have to travel to the rational part of the brain, but first they have to go through the limbic system. Emotions are largely housed in the limbic system, and it has a great deal to do with the formation of memories. What this means is that we have an emotional reaction to situations, first, before we start rationalizing. Mary was letting the Baltimore riots affect her because she was only letting things through her RAS on what she believed based on the memories of her son, and her limbic system was replaying those emotions.

How do resilient individuals manage their negative emotions and feel appreciation at the same time? How do they implement that REFRAME button?

Your reticular activating system is the center of control for other parts of the brain involved in learning, self-control, and motivation. Like a filter between your conscious mind and your subconscious mind, it takes instructions from your conscious mind and passes them on to your subconscious. For example, when you are at an airport, there is so much information coming to you, yet your ears perk up when you hear your flight number being called out. Why? Because you trained your RAS to pay attention to and filter only *that* information rather than all the other announcements and nearby conversations from fellow travellers.

Similarly, neuroscience has shown that you can condition your RAS to new filters of information, thereby creating a growth mindset rather than a stagnant mindset. When resilient individuals appreciate what they have rather than what they don't have, they have conditioned their RAS to look for that information and process it at the same time as facing challenges. My mother has trained her RAS to filter information to appreciate what she already has that other people may not have. Your RAS is like a radar detector; it will only bring through information that you want to give attention to or feel aroused by.

You've read books or gone to seminars where the author or speaker has told you to make a list of goals and read them every day or visualize them. The reason for that is because you're training your RAS to help you detect information that will help you achieve your goals. Hence, your RAS is your REFRAME button, which you must train to look for the things you have and appreciate rather than feel pity for what you don't have. This kind of training will help you get out of the rut of worrying about challenges and instead to champion those challenges into lessons and opportunities.

Here are some tools that can help train your RAS to look for appreciation:

1. Meditate for 5 to 15 minutes every day and appreciate the things you already have and the lessons you've learned from all your challenges.

2. At the end of the year, on December 30, write 10 accomplishments you've had and put it up somewhere. I have mine on the inside of one of my office cupboards.

3. At the beginning of the year, On January 1, write 10 goals (big or small) you'd like to accomplish that year and put it up somewhere.

4. Bless your competition because they're keeping you from becoming complacent.

5. Appreciate one little thing every day while you drive or while taking a shower.

Chapter 16

Beliefs

It's not the load that breaks you down; it's the way you carry it.

— Lena Horne

A belief is what you hold to be true and what shapes your reality. As my mentor Tim Hallbom explains: "A belief is an idea that expresses meaning for you. It's a way of describing what causes certain life situations for you, as well as what's possible for you." Similarly, you may hold beliefs about the world, such as "doing sales is sleazy," "women are weak leaders," or "I'm not organized." Someone else may hold a different belief, such as "making sales is meeting others' needs," "women make great leaders," or "I'm organized and efficient."

When I coached clients on releasing weight, one of the most common beliefs I heard was, "It's too much work to lose weight." Sure enough, these same individuals had previously been on other weight loss programs where coming off of their routine eating behaviours and creating new eating behaviours and food sacrifices caused more work, which they deemed too strenuous. A healthy lifestyle approach is

159

not just about changing the foods one eats; it's also about changing beliefs and behaviours.

Beliefs guide our behaviour and then **we expect** something to happen because we believe it will. This has been proven in many medical studies where participating patients have been administered a placebo. However, these patients believe they are being cured and act as if (behaviour) the drug is a miracle; thus, the patient's health improves (expectancy). Vlad Dolezal says it best: **"A belief is your best explanation of the world,** *based on your current evidence.*"

In India, elephants are tied to a wooden post with a rope to keep them from running away from their owners. In Kenya, where I grew up, we were scared of elephants because these beasts could kill a person. Yet, one might wonder, what would keep grown elephants tied to a wooden post? Elephant trainers in India explain that when a baby elephant is born, the trainer ties it to the post with a rope and even though the elephant tries to get away, the rope is stronger. In time the baby elephant comes to believe that it cannot escape the rope; therefore, it learns that when it is tied, escape is futile. However, this elephant grows up into a beast and can easily break free of the rope, but it doesn't believe it can because that learning was ingrained into its belief system.

160

How many people are held back by a rope and believe they can't bounce back? Our beliefs start forming at the age of three, and most of our core beliefs are formed between the ages of six and eight. Core beliefs are the way we see ourselves, others, and the world around us. The baby elephant forms a core belief that it cannot escape, and it carries this core belief into adulthood. You have core beliefs that you hold tightly to, and you tend to focus on information that supports these beliefs rather than contradicts them. Most beliefs are under the surface, and we can't see them because they make up our understanding.

Robert Dilts and Tim and Kris Hallbom, leaders in neuro linguistic programming (NLP), have identified four types of subconscious limiting beliefs that keep you from having what you want. The first step toward changing these limiting beliefs is to learn how to identify them and become consciously aware of them. The next step is to change these limiting beliefs into empowering ones, so you can start positively transforming your life and business. As you read through these four types of subconscious limiting beliefs, start identifying your own:

1. **Beliefs about cause:** These beliefs usually have the word "because" in them, and you believe there is a

specific cause creating the belief. Some examples include:

a) I can't do public speaking because I stutter.

b) I can't be successful in business because I wouldn't know how to run it, and my parents were unsuccessful.

c) Too much wealth is the cause of family problems.

2. **Beliefs about meaning:** We try to find meaning in almost everything. For example, what does it mean when a salesperson in the company has acquired the highest sales again? Does it mean the salesperson is lucky, or does it mean this salesperson works hard? The meaning that one puts behind these beliefs will guide behaviour because that is all you filter through. Some examples include:

a) Being a woman means you have to work harder.

b) Too much wealth makes people behave differently.

c) Change is very challenging.

3. **Beliefs about possibility:** These beliefs are about what is possible and are broken down further into categories:

a) **The outcome is possible.** If the outcome is possible, then you will go for the desired outcome.

b) **The outcome is impossible.** If it is impossible, then you will not bother trying to go for the outcome and you will give up ahead of time. Some examples include:

    i. Starting a business in this economy is impossible.

    ii. The doctor has said I only have a few months to live.

    iii. This project goes beyond our scope.

4. **Beliefs about identity:** These beliefs are more about worthiness and they circle around success. Some examples include:

a) I'm not worthy of success.

b) I'm not smart enough to be successful.

c) I don't have it in me to be resilient.

People who know me ask how I managed to overcome my speech impediment, or how I lived halfway across the world without my parents or how I managed to get nominated as Business of the Year in my town in only our fourth year. As I look back, I realize that I used a process to blow out the limiting belief and replace it with a new, empowering belief.

This process is also commonly used in NLP and includes the following steps:

1. Identify a limiting belief. For the longest time in my life, I believed that I'd never be able to do any presentations or public speaking.

2. Identify the supportive evidence. I'd get nervous in school and not be able to get out a sentence. I thought people who stutter couldn't speak in public because it's too difficult.

3. Identify the positive intention or secondary gain of this belief. What is the payoff of believing in this limiting belief? The payoff is, I'd still have friends and not be different; Keeps me from feeling embarrassed or stupid.

4. Take the evidence from item 2 and counter it so that it no longer supports the limiting belief.

   - Evidence 1: Gets nervous in school and cannot get a word out during presentations.

   - Re-framed evidence: I didn't practice my presentation enough, and I could have practiced with family members.

   - Evidence 2: I stuttered and people who stutter cannot speak in public.

- Re-frame evidence: There are many famous people who stutter.

Weaken this limiting belief even more by asking these questions:

What would my mentor tell me about this limiting belief?

What kind of behaviours will I continue to have if I continue holding on to this limiting belief?

5. State your new well-formed belief, which is usually the opposite of your limiting belief. For example: I can speak easily and manage my fears about it.

6. Find evidence to support this new well-formed belief so that it completely squashes the old limiting belief. For example:

   - When I practice the presentation and use my fluency skills, I feel more confident, like getting an A in a product development presentation in university or the time I presented my public health case to my colleagues.

   - I have been able to speak easily in other situations that I thought I couldn't before.

The idea of this process is to diminish the emotional charge that the old limiting belief has by finding counter evidence that doesn't support it. As you work on affirming your new, well-formed belief, you will find more evidence as you go along in life to support it!

PART 3 – Three Steps to Building Your Resilience Reflex

Chapter 17

Release

Learn to get in touch with the silence within yourself and know that everything in life has a purpose.

– Elisabeth Kubler-Ross

In 2011, George S. Everly, executive director of Resiliency Sciences Institutes at the University of Maryland, was asked, "What's the difference between those who choose to sink or swim in times of adversity?" He stated two factors:

1. A lack of perspective stemming from inadequate preparation and tenacity.
2. A negative attitude.

He further explained that resilience can be taught and self-esteem can be earned through personal accomplishment in the face of a challenge.

In my 3-step method you will gain some tools on building that resilience muscle, which is in atrophy now. As you practice this 3-step method, you will notice your resilience muscle getting stronger so that in times of challenge, crisis, meltdowns, or a demanding environment, the practice of resilience becomes your first reflex.

Just as individuals build their resilience muscle and achieve self-efficacy, so too can organizations develop a culture of resilience, but that comes from having resilient leaders who have certain traits and continually invest in their employees and clients and encourage innovation.

What is involved in becoming a resilient leader? The answer is in Everly's statement above: having a positive attitude and proper preparation to have enough perspective to bounce back. Earlier in the book, I discussed the 5 keys to building a positive attitude. Let's turn to how one can prepare to get unstuck from a challenge by changing perspective.

As noted earlier, my mother lost nearly everything at the age of 66, but now she appreciates life and is paying her debts. When I visited my mother in Kenya as she was going through this crisis, she couldn't stop crying, and her thoughts revolved around being stuck where she was—in debt, broken, and hurt emotionally. At that time, I told her something that to this day she tells me is the cause of her getting unstuck and bouncing back. I recall being in her kitchen making some Kenyan tea for breakfast and having a conversation, when she started crying again. She kept bringing up things from the past or how things had turned out.

"Can you hear yourself?" I asked her. "I know you are going through a tough time, and I couldn't even imagine going through it at your age, but all I hear is you living in the past hurt rather than trying to move forward. What has happened has happened, and you can't change it. Do you want to continue with these kinds of thoughts in your head that make you feel miserable? Because the mother I know has always taught me to find a way," I said.

There is a place for negative thoughts, and as human beings, we tend to let our emotions guide our thoughts because that is the way we are programmed. I'm not indicating that one has to think positively all the time. In fact, it's fine to think negatively at first, as long as you recognize and become aware that at some point (and quickly) one must press the STOP button on those negative tapes and insert positive tapes and press PLAY.

Resilient leaders and organizations cannot afford to play those negative tapes because it hurts their bottom line and affects the work culture. So where does one start to get unstuck and hit the RELEASE button? In my research, I have found that resilient individuals and leaders use at least one of these 3 tools to get unstuck, and I call this process RELEASE:

1. Becoming aware of their thoughts, words, and feelings in order to change their results.
2. The code—they have a unique phrase, which opens up the door to possibility.
3. The circle of resilience, which involves stepping into powerful emotional states on demand.

Becoming Aware of Our Words

My mentor and coach, Michael Losier, author of *Law of Attraction: The Science of Attracting More of What You Want and Less of What You Don't*, explains how our words affect our thoughts, and our thoughts affect our feelings. The law of attraction matches those feelings and gives you more of the same back. Therefore, if you are feeling negative, the universal law will match that feeling and give more negative results in your life. However, if you don't believe in the law of attraction and look at this logically, you will realize that when you say negative things or think negative thoughts, you will end up feeling negative and therefore you will behave in that manner, causing negative results in your life.

For example, I recently spoke to a well-known volunteer organization that has been around for 100 years and is experiencing a lot of change. Some leaders who have been with the organization for years are resisting change, whereas some are all for change because they believe it will bring in new members with fresh perspectives. Here are some things I heard said by those who resisted change; notice how words affect thoughts, feelings, and results:

Words: I don't like the changes taking place in our organization.

Thoughts: We're going to lose our identity; this will lead to chaos; we can't afford to bring in changes now.

Feelings: anxiety, regret, guilt (all negative feelings)

Behaviors/Results: lack of continuity; lack of new members enrolling; more chaos and conflict.

To change your results, you have to work backwards.

In order to feel positive, you have to think positively, but in order to think positively, one must use positive words.

Whenever you catch yourself thinking or saying the words **DON'T, NOT or NO**, ask yourself, "So what do I (we) want?" Make sure your answer is stated in the positive and starts with, "I want…"

This organization changed their words to, "We want a sustainable organization." As soon as that happened, the members subconsciously released themselves from being stuck in chaos and moved ahead to overcoming the challenges they faced.

The Code

After interviewing and reading about resilient individuals who have gone through personal and professional challenges, I have noticed that the way they release or get unstuck is by using a subconscious phrase. For example,

1. Horror author J. Thorn's phrase is, "No matter how bad it seems, there's always an opportunity."

2. Former child soldier and now musician and philanthropist Emmanuel Jal uses a phrase, "Shine light where there's darkness."

3. Olympic athlete Louis Zamperini's consistent phrase while he practiced for his races, got stuck in a raft for 47 days, and was held captive in a war camp was, "You have to be prepared."

When I find myself faced with a challenge, my phrase is, "There's a way; what is that way?" I call this a code because it's unique to each person. This code allows me to dominate negative feelings and fires me up to get back on track. Do you have a code to fire you up?

Create a code that you can use in times of adversity. Use that code when you feel your back is against the wall or when you think you have run out of options; you will be surprised by what happens next.

The Circle of Resilience

This technique is adapted from the behavioural modeling work of Richard Bandler and John Grinder, who found that people who are exceptional at what they do are able to step into the right mental state for the right activity at the right time. This technique would be beneficial in creating a mental state of resilience during times of adversity or change, but like with everything, you have to practice:

1. Think of a specific situation where you were going through some challenge and you weren't as resilient as you would have liked to be.

2. Standing up, imagine an invisible circle on the floor directly in front you. Make this circle large enough to walk into, and use your imagination to notice the color, brightness, and any other details about it. This is your circle, so add anything you want to make it positive for you. For example, when I'm preparing to speak on stage, I step into a golden circle that spirals up and around me.

3. Think of an emotion you'd like to have, such as resilience or mental toughness. Now think of a time in your life when you felt that strong sense of resilience.

4. Go back to that moment or time where you felt that resilient emotion and relive or re-experience that mental state, and as you do that, step inside the circle. Use your senses to FEEL this state and FEEL it in your body, too. Feel that powerful emotion surrounding you and flowing through your body. Breathe in the feeling and enjoy it fully.

5. Now think of a cue that will remind you to step into your circle (one that seems related to the state), so that you can access this powerful emotion for resilience. This cue could be a phrase, a word, or a hand gesture. It is important to do this because it automatically reminds you to step into the circle and demand a positive emotional state.

6. Before the intensity of the feeling fades, step out of the circle to return to a neutral state.

7. Repeat the steps a few more times by stepping into your circle and imagining yourself in the future during the time that you need to feel resilient—a week, a month, or even a year from now. Visualize yourself stepping into the circle on your cue and

175

accessing that powerful emotional state of resilience when you need it.

BONUS: Use this same circle to access other positive emotional states like creativity, clarity, humor, efficiency, and so on.

Chapter 18

Reprogram

Our greatest weakness lies in giving up. The most certain way to succeed is always to try just one more time.

— Thomas Edison

The second step in becoming more resilient involves re-programming ourselves to find solutions. You are releasing old patterns and reprogramming new skill sets, and as Donald Meichanbaum, Ph.D., of the Melissa Institute states, "Resilience develops from everyday magic of ordinary resources. Resilience is not a sign of exceptional strength, but a fundamental feature of normal, everyday coping skills."

In Dr. Meichanbaum's report, *Important Facts About Resilience: A Consideration Of Research Findings About Resilience and Implications For Assessment and Treatment*, he points out that most spouses of returning military service members believe that deployment strengthened their marriages. Only 10 percent believed that deployment weakened their union. Deployment contributed to the development of new family skills and competencies and instilled a sense of independence, confidence, and problem-solving skills.

177

When there are challenges and changes to face, re-programming a new skill set becomes necessary. This is evident now more than ever with new technology emerging faster than most can keep up. Yet, we have shown that we can adapt. When the first cell phone was released, we were all intrigued because it meant that we could have a phone outside our homes. Then smart phones were introduced, where not only can a person call another, but also connect with messaging and email via the internet. This meant we now have a mini computer and phone in a single device. Notably, this occurred only within the last 20 years. The human brain is like a problem-solving machine, and it's extremely creative, yet we limit ourselves to that creativity by our own beliefs about what is possible.

During the 3-year period from 2009 to 2012, my husband's 20-year old retail clothing store was losing money. The retail industry was changing, and the economy had tanked after the 2008 financial crisis. At that time, I didn't have much to do with the business, but I did know he was borrowing equity from our home to pay suppliers. In 2011, we sat down to assess our situation because we couldn't continue paying for a business that was dragging us to bankruptcy. The business was in debt by $220,000! We had purchased a home in 2001 and a mortgage of only $50,000 remained, so we decided to refinance our home. In the summer of 2012, we hired an auction company to auction what was left of the merchandise, and we officially closed the retail store; we then paid off our debts and successfully avoided bankruptcy.

Being in so much debt was no fun because we literally felt stuck with our backs against the wall. A part of me kept blaming my husband, especially for the fact that we had to re-mortgage our house when we were so close to paying it off. Another part of me was glad, though, that we had a found a solution without compromising our livelihood or marriage.

Most of us are stuck in the "blame mindset" when we are faced with challenges. In this mindset, you may catch yourself saying things, such as the following:

- Why do I have this problem?
- How long will I have this problem?
- Whose fault is it that I have this problem?
- What's wrong?

When you use this questioning method, you are taking up a "blame mindset" because you will still feel oppressed and broken and that you lack choices. However, it is possible to re-program yourself to an "outcome mindset" by asking alternative questions, such as these:

- What do I want and when do I want it?

- When I get what I want, what else in my life will improve?

- What resources do I have available to help me with this challenge?

- Can I utilize these resources to the best of my ability or do I require extra help?

- What can I do now to improve this situation and get what I want?

Having an outcome mindset propels a person toward critical questioning, where you start thinking of solutions right away. It also provides the feeling of relief and hope as you start generating ideas.

In previous chapters, I offered a glimpse of how I used re-programming in different areas of my life to overcome personal and business obstacles, from moving to a new country, to overcoming my speech impediment and releasing my struggles with weight, to working through business challenges at the wellness centre and building my training business. However, I'm always asked how I did it or how I balanced it all. The truth is, I've trained myself to have an outcome mindset, but I've also used two extra strategies to help re-program new skill sets and to easily bounce back. These strategies were previously shared in chapter 10 but will be outlined in detail; these principles can be used alone or in combination, depending on how far you've come in finding solutions:

1. Mentor Magic: Resilient individuals use this technique subconsciously to get information that they may not have considered. This is another way of improving your decision-making and problem solving skills.

2. Future Reading (without a psychic): This is where you step into the future and see your problem solved and then look back to see what steps you took to solve that problem.

Mentor Magic (adapted from Tim Hallbom, NLP Institute of California)

1. Identify a situation in which you are unsure about what steps to take or what decision to make.

2. Think of 2 to 3 mentors whom you know that will give you honest feedback and who will believe in you. Choose mentors that may have been in the same context that you are in, but who inspire you.

3. Stand up and place your imaginary mentors around you. If it helps, get pieces of colored paper and write the mentor's name on a piece of paper; repeat that

for the other papers. Place these papers on the floor around you.

4. Step into one mentor and become that mentor in mind and body. Give yourself a message on the situation you are unsure about or are stuck at.

5. Now step out of the mentor and listen to the message again, coming from your mentor this time as yourself.

6. Repeat steps 4 and 5 for the other mentors you've chosen.

7. After you've heard the messages, figure out the common advice they are giving you and go for it.

I use different mentors for different situations, and I encourage you to do the same. When I'm about to speak on stage, I place two imaginary mentors on stage with me that are awesome at pumping energy and humor into the room. When I'm coaching, I imagine my coaches who taught me, sitting next to me and guiding me. Make a list of mentors with whom you identify in different contexts.

Future Reading (without consulting a psychic): An NLP Process

1. Imagine a straight line in front of you that starts at your current state and goes into the future to a

specific time where your problem has been solved, for example, three months, six months, or a year.

2. Pay attention to your physiology as you walk from where you are to the time on your line where the problem has been solved.

3. Choose your pace and notice what you feel, hear, and see.

4. When you get to the space on the line where your problem is solved, stop and turn around completely to look back towards the current state (present) and ask yourself, "How did this get solved? What did I do to get to a solution?"

5. Take note of any ideas that come to mind and say them out loud so you can hear them.

6. When you are done, walk back to the current state (present) smiling and feeling accomplished.

As you embrace and practice these new skill sets in helping you problem-solve and make decisions, you will find that solutions come more easily and your productivity enhances. This is when you become a master problem solver, which is a great sign of resiliency.

Chapter 19

Resolve

The ultimate measure of a man is not where he stands in moments of comfort and convenience, but where he stands in time of challenge and controversy.

— Dr. Martin Luther King, Jr.

Resolve is the third step in my process toward building your resilience reflex in life and business. This step involves taking action, having cognitive flexibility, and mastering yourself in the process. Across history, certain figures have demonstrated the utmost in resilience, especially when a country, culture, or religious sect is working against that individual's values and principles. These figures include Jesus Christ, Mahatma Gandhi, Martin Luther King, Malcolm X, Nelson Mandela, and others.

How did these individuals manage their emotions and create a positive attitude? How did they re-program themselves and bounce back time after time, even when they felt they couldn't put any more effort into their cause? What kept them motivated to take action, to keep trying, and to never quit? The answer is simple: They believed.

Our limiting beliefs and fears stop us from taking action, but if one believes in a cause, an idea, or project, nothing will get in the way of getting it off the ground. If you have doubts, then re-read the chapter on beliefs to help work through those reservations. However, another common problem in taking action is a lack of motivation, which occurs for three different reasons:

1. You are using words that don't support your action. For example, you think you "should" or you "must" instead of "I will" or "I'm going to."
2. You feel overwhelmed with the task ahead of you. I felt that way when I started writing this book and when I started my business, but I broke things down into smaller tasks or parts so I could manage and feel more motivated to take action.
3. There isn't enough to motivate you, so think about the benefit you will get or how you will feel when the task is done. This feeling of achievement will propel you to take action.

There will be times that you want to give up or slide back to your old habits. Acknowledge that part of you and understand the subconscious messages your body is sending you. I know I have felt like giving up at certain times. Why can't I be like a normal person who is happy working eight hours a day, enjoys vacations, enjoys the benefits, and retires with a good pension? Because I'm not normal! I am extraordinary, I am a difference-maker, I am a knowledge seeker and giver and I'm a guide. I know that when I'm mentally exhausted, I tend to want to give up, but I have learned how to take a mental break, how to delegate, and refocus again. As you practice this 3-step system, start recognizing when you feel this way and come up with ways you can deal with it.

Between 2009 and 2010, when I was completing my master's in neuro linguistic programming, one of the main topics we were learned was *modelling motivation*. I found out that successful people have this same system of motivating themselves and the steps include:

1. You have a task, and it may be unpleasant. For example, cleaning the house is the example I chose in the class.
2. Say to yourself, "It will feel great when the task (cleaning the house) is done."
3. Visualize the task (cleaning the house) completed or being accomplished. Here I'd visualize my home sparkly clean, organized and easy to find things again.

4. Access the feeling of seeing the task completed (I felt good and proud of having an organized home) and stay in that good feeling.

5. Say to yourself in a positive tone, "Now go do it."

After becoming aware of this motivation strategy, I noticed that I used this for physical exercise, for creating products, for project work or deadlines, and for mundane tasks like filing and cooking.

It seems pretty easy to comprehend, but still most procrastinate even after we have gone through the first two steps – Release and Re-program. Remember, you don't have to do everything either, you can delegate or outsource tasks within a task. For example, one of my goals was to convert my behavioural weight loss book into an audio book and find a site that would host the audio tracks. The project seemed overwhelming because I thought I had to go to the studio, record, edit, and upload the files. I had never done this before, and I did not want to pay hundreds of dollars either. I decided to outsource the editing and uploading by finding a freelancer on *Upwork,* and the person I hired taught me to use a free program on my Mac laptop to record my book. I recorded my book over three mornings, uploaded the files to *Dropbox*, and he did the rest, which involved editing and hosting the audio tracks on a site where I already have a membership.

This task seemed overwhelming at first, but as soon as I broke it down into smaller parts, utilized the resources I had, and outsourced the rest, I got motivated to take action and complete my audio book. I was also being flexible in my approach to this task. Instead of giving up and saying to myself, "This is too much work, costs a lot money, I don't have time, and it has to be perfect," I found a way to make this easier for myself, and in the process I ended up with another product at a minimal personal price.

Flexibility in decision-making is important because it allows you to change strategies when necessary.

You've heard the phrase, "You can take a horse to the water, but you cannot force it to drink." I have shared many tools and strategies in this book to help you build your resilience muscle, but it's up to you to practice and take action. In other words, I'm giving you an equipped gym bag, and I'm driving you to the gym, but in the end you have to lift the weights. You will start first with lighter weights, but as you get stronger and build muscles, you will move on to heavier weights; as you do that, you feel more confident about your health, you feel good, and you are training your body to be resilient even though lifting heavier weights will strain your muscles and cause soreness.

I'm certainly not the same person I was 15 years ago. I worked at finding my voice, my confidence, and my worth. There were times that I did not want to step outside the comfort I knew and when I did, it caused pain and anxiety (just like having sore muscles), but I did it anyway because it was important to me. The more I step into the very real possibility that I hold the key to my freedom to choose, create and live, the more exciting life becomes. What is important to you? Now go do it!

Access your bonus gift.

Enjoy this BONUS gift immediately:

A workbook based on the 3-step system found in this book.

Visit http://www.zaheennanji.com/rrbook to access this BONUS gift now!

THE
RESILIENCE
REFLEX

WORKBOOK

3 Powerful Steps to Get Unstuck and Bounce Back

ZAHEEN NANJI

References

Loiser, Michael. 2007. *Law of Attraction – the Science of Attracting More of What you Want and Less of What you Don't.* Hatchette Book Group

McKenna, Paul. 2009. *Control Stress: Stop Worrying and Feel Good Now.* Bantam Press.

O'Connor, Joseph. 2005. *Free Yourself from Fears.* Nicholas Brealey Publishing.

Ready, Romilla; Kate Burton. 2004. *Neuro Linguistic Programming for Dummies.* John Wiley & Sons Ltd.

Reivich, Karen; Schatte, Andrew Ph.D. 2003. *The Resilience Factor: 7 Keys to Finding Your Inner Strength and Overcoming Life's Hurdles.* Broadway Books, A Division of Random House.

Wiseman, Richard. 2013. *Rip It Up: The Radically New Approach to Changing Your Life.* MacMillan.

Davis-Laack, Paula M.A.P.P. 2014, October 2. *Seven Things Resilient Employees Do Differently.* Psychology Today.

Henderson, Nan. 2007. *Hard-Wired to Bounce Back.* Resiliency in Action.

Meichenbaum, Donald Ph.D. n.d. *Important Facts About Resilience: A Consideration of Research Findings About Resilience and Implications for Assessment and Treatment.* Melissa Institute , Miami, Florida

SVYASA – a Yoga Research Organization. 2007. What are the Effects of Laughter Yoga on Stress in the Workplace? Laughter Yoga International.

The Resilience Inventory: Seven Essential Skills for Overcoming Life's Obstacles and Determining Happiness, Vol. 20, No. 6. 2004, December. Selection & Development Review.

The Road to Resilience Guide. n.d. American Psychological Association.

What is Contemporary Stress? 2006, Spring. Institute of Heart Math Newsletter.

Certified Training in Masters Neuro Linguistic Programming - NLP Institute of California: www.nlpca.com

Certified Training in Wealthy Mind Training by Tim and Kris Hallbom: http://thewealthymind.com

http://en.wikipedia.org/wiki/2015_Baltimore_protests
http://vladdolezal.com/blog/latest/page/16

http://www.biography.com/people/louis-zamperini

http://www.reticularactivatingsystem.org

About the Author

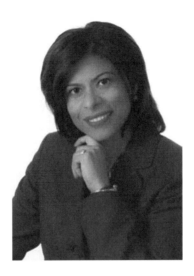

People who don't know Zaheen's background sometimes assume that achieving success was easy for her. That couldn't be further from the truth. Her first challenge began around age 5, when an incident left her with a speech impediment-stuttering. As she got accustomed to the people around her in Kenya and they got accustomed to her speech, another change occurred at the age of 15 - her parents sent her to Canada to create better educational opportunities, but this move made her speech even worse; she lost confidence in herself and found comfort in food. Even after going through speech therapy in her twenties, Zaheen wasn't cured, but this was the stepping stone to finding her VOICE.

As Zaheen completed her education in Nutrition & Food Science and Environmental Health, she became determined to understand the source of her speech impediment because it had such an impact on things she wanted to do but felt she couldn't. Using her strategies to embrace fear rather than run from it, she slowly started her transformation.

While balancing her family, Zaheen has created a successful health and wellness business and simultaneously acquired 3 rental properties within a span of less than 36 months. Not only an entrepreneur and small business owner, Zaheen is also the author of an award-winning book on behavior weight loss which won a bronze medal at the Global E-book Awards and was featured in the top 10 in Women Business Owners Today E-zine . Her system of transformation and excellence is grounded in building your resilience muscle which is the daily practice of the three R's - Release, Reprogram and Resolve. She offers an array of time-tested techniques and powerful principles to propel her clients toward their definitions of success.

WEBSITE
http://www.zaheennanji.com